The New Zealand Dyslexia Handbook

Tom Nicholson and Susan Dymock

NZCER PRESS

Wellington 2015

NZCER PRESS
New Zealand Council for Educational Research
PO Box 3237
Wellington
New Zealand

© Tom Nicholson and Susan Dymock, 2015

ISBN 978-1-927231-44-9

This book is copyright 2015 by NZCER Press.

This book is not a photocopiable master.

No part of the publication may be copied, stored or communicated in any form by any means (paper or digital), including recording or storing in an electronic retrieval system, without the written permission of the publisher.
Education institutions that hold a current licence with Copyright Licensing New Zealand, may copy from this book in strict accordance with the terms of the CLNZ Licence.

A catalogue record for this book is available from the National Library of New Zealand

Designed by Cluster Creative, Wellington
Cover artwork by Timon Maxey
Printed by About Print, Wellington

Distributed by NZCER Distribution Services
PO Box 3237
Wellington
New Zealand
www.nzcer.org.nz

Dedication

We dedicate this book to the late Professor Emeritus and Professor on Recall, Robert Calfee, of Stanford University, who has inspired us over many years with his amazing insights into reading and spelling, and his passion to change our teaching of literacy for the better.

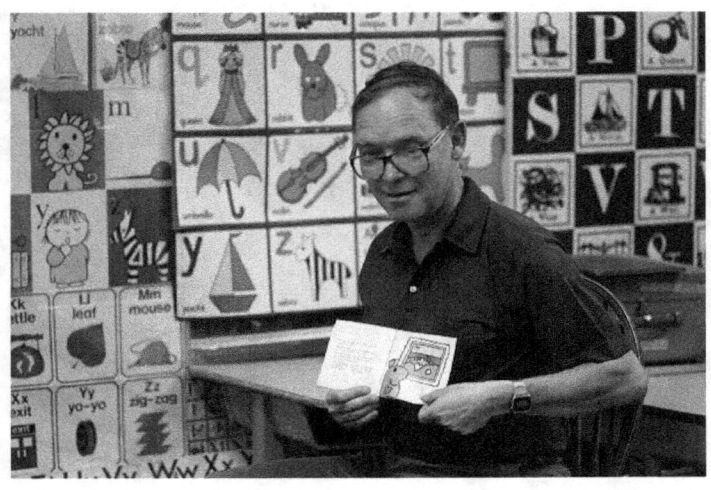

Acknowledgements

The video, *Talking about Dyslexia*, which accompanies this book was funded by the ANZ Bank Staff Foundation, the Faculty of Education at the University of Waikato, and Chris Reeve, a private donor. We are really grateful for this support.

A special thank you to Esperance, William, Ryan and their families who shared their dyslexia stories for the video. We also thank Fiona Bradley, Principal, Tauwhare School, and Loveday, William's Year 8 teacher, for their insight into dyslexia-friendly schools and classrooms.

Thanks to the many children and parents we have worked with over the years in our university after-school reading centres for inspiring us to write about dyslexia. Thanks to David Ellis of NZCER Press, for his faith in the book. Thanks to Sumner Schachter for reading the manuscript and giving ideas about "dot-to-dot" phonics, to Mary Delahunty for the list of apps in Chapter 9, and to Laura Tse for sharing her lessons on Big Book reading. Thanks to Professors Michael Corbalis, Elena Grigorenko, and Max Coltheart for reviewing Chapter 1, "What is Dyslexia". A final thanks to our families for their support and allowing us the many hours of time at home while we worked on the book.

Contents

Dedication		iii
Acknowledgements		v
Introduction		1
PART ONE	**Getting to know dyslexia**	9
Chapter 1	What is dyslexia?	11
Chapter 2	Misconceptions about dyslexia	23
PART TWO	**Living with dyslexia**	27
Chapter 3	Dyslexia, family and the school	29
Chapter 4	Dyslexia, self-esteem and behaviour	37
PART THREE	**Assessing dyslexia**	47
Chapter 5	Dyslexia and the simple view of reading and writing	49
Chapter 6	Screening for dyslexia	57
PART FOUR	**Tackling dyslexia**	77
Chapter 7	Teaching children with dyslexia to read	79
Chapter 8	Teaching pupils with dyslexia to spell and write	121
Chapter 9	The importance of fluency and how to teach it effectively	139
Chapter 10	Making the classroom a dyslexia-friendly place	149
PART FIVE	**Final word**	161
Chapter 11	A final word	163

APPENDICES:	**Resources**	167
Appendix 1	Assessment measures	169
Appendix 1A	Burt Word Reading Test	170
Appendix 1B	Bryant Test of Basic Decoding Skills	175
Appendix 1C	Alphabet Test	178
Appendix 1D	GKR Phonemic Awareness Test	181
Appendix 1E	Invented Spelling Test	185
Appendix 2	Edward Fry's 200 common words, in order of frequency	187
Appendix 3	Lesson plans for teaching children with dyslexia to read	188
	(a) Short *e* vowel	186
	(b) Consonant *y*	189
	(c) Consonant blend *st*	191
	(d) Long vowel sound *i*	193
	(e) Vowel digraph *oa*	195
	(f) Open and closed syllables	196
Appendix 4	Spelling activities	201
	(a) Practice for phonemic awareness—turtle talk	199
	(b) Dot-to-dot phonics	200
	(c) Phonics strips	201
	(d) Sound boxes	203
Appendix 5	Phonogram charts	205
Appendix 6	A spelling programme to teach Anglo-Saxon vowel spelling patterns	208
Appendix 7	Examples of individual spelling tutoring	245
Appendix 8	Lesson plans combining Big Book reading and explicit phonics to help with spelling	251
Appendix 9	Questionnaire for students	257
References		259
Glossary		269
Index		275

Introduction

Bridging the knowledge gap

In this book and accompanying video clips* we aim to raise awareness about dyslexia, because it remains largely mysterious and misunderstood in schools and the community. For example, a British survey of the general public (Whitehead, 2007), polling 1,000 adults, found that three-quarters understood little or nothing about dyslexia, one in five thought that dyslexics just need to work harder, and half thought dyslexia is just getting words and letters back to front. The survey also asked the general public if they thought they had dyslexia, and 1 percent thought they did. This might well be an underestimate given that so many did not know much about dyslexia.

On the positive side, in New Zealand dyslexia was officially recognised by the Ministry of Education in 2007, and New Zealand schools seem to be knowledgeable about dyslexia. We did our own survey of schools and found (see Chapter 3) that nearly all schools surveyed believed they had students with dyslexia. On the negative side, fewer than half of the schools felt skilled enough to teach these students.

Much research has been done on dyslexia, but this information is not always filtering through to where it is needed most. This book aims to bridge the gap between research on dyslexia and school and community understanding. It provides readers with answers to questions we are often asked, such as:

- What is dyslexia?
- What does the latest research tell us about the brain and dyslexia?
- How do I know if one of my students has dyslexia?

* *Talking About Dyslexia*, see www.nzcer.org.nz/nzcerpress/new-zealand-dyslexia-handbook.

- How do I screen for dyslexia?
- How do I teach students with dyslexia to read and spell?
- How do I go about making my classroom dyslexia friendly?

An introduction to dyslexia

What is dyslexia?

What is dyslexia? The word *dyslexia* is derived from Greek. If we break it into its two meaningful parts, *dys* + *lexia*, we have *difficulty* + *words*, or difficulty with words. Dyslexia means difficulty with words, particularly printed words. Dyslexia is also unexpected in the sense that students who have dyslexia are not the ones parents and teachers normally think would have trouble reading words. So the simple answer to 'What is dyslexia?' is that dyslexia is an unexpected difficulty with reading and writing. It is unexpected in the sense that students with dyslexia seem to be average or better in terms of their general ability, especially their spoken language, and yet they struggle with reading and spelling.

How long have we known about dyslexia?

Dyslexia has been known about for more than 100 years. In November 1896 the *British Medical Journal* published what experts consider to be the first reference to developmental dyslexia; that is, reading difficulty that has occurred in the normal course of growing up and is not due to trauma, such as a car accident (Shaywitz, 1996). B. Pringle Morgan, a British general practitioner, refers to Percy F., a 14-year-old boy, who "has always been a bright and intelligent boy, quick at games, and in no way inferior to others of his age. His great difficulty has been—and is now—his inability to learn to read" (Morgan, 1896, p. 1378). Morgan continues, "The greatest efforts have been made to teach him to read, but in spite of this laborious and persistent training, he can only with difficulty spell out words of one syllable." Well over a century later students like Percy can still be found in primary and secondary classrooms. Those with dyslexia are our neighbours, friends, fathers, mothers, sons, daughters, aunts, uncles, nieces and nephews.

Are students with dyslexia that way because their parents neglected them?

Students with dyslexia are not usually from a poor or neglected home background. To give an example from our own experience, both of us ran after-school university reading centres for many years, focusing on struggling readers and writers. Sue still does run a centre because she has always been able to find sponsorship to offer free lessons. Tom had sponsorship for a while but then had to charge a small fee.

When a fee was charged there was a dramatic change in clientele. The parents who were poor almost all dropped out. The remaining children were still struggling with reading, but one day we realised their parents were almost all middle class and European. Children were not arriving on foot anymore, but in BMWs, yet they had dyslexia. This is why dyslexia is surprising. Our after-school pupils were not disabled or disadvantaged. They went to good schools and came from well-off, loving homes. They were struggling with literacy for no other reason than that they could not 'crack the code'.

Dyslexia in today's digital world

Today, compared to 1896 when dyslexia was first written about, we are surrounded by print. Students use cell phones, smart phones, tablets, computers, newspapers and magazines, in addition to the school reading material they encounter for hours every day. It seems impossible for most of us to survive without the Internet, yet many of our children will struggle to be able to enter this new digital world unless we do something now.

What does it feel like to have dyslexia?

As revealed in the video clips that accompany this book, dyslexic students feel frustrated at not being able to do what their classmates can do, and this frustration is shared by their parents. They desperately search for more time to do their work at school because it takes them so much longer, but the school clock is unable to wait for them. They are anxious about not being able to meet national standards. William reported not sleeping well, his parents reported him tugging on his lips as a physical sign of anxiousness. This is not good.

It is not surprising these students feel frustrated, isolated, lonely and 'dumb'. How do students with dyslexia feel when they are 'pulled out' in front of their peers to attend Reading Recovery or some other remedial programme? Imagine if your classmates teased you, or called you dumb, because of your difficulty with reading and writing. What's more, imagine if, when you were called to go to remedial reading, it was at a time when you were engaged in the subjects you enjoyed and excelled in (e.g., a science experiment, mathematics, or art).

The video clips that accompany this book: insights into dyslexia

Once you watch the video clips that accompany this book you will know what we mean when we say dyslexia often surprises us. The two boys interviewed, William and Ryan, are very articulate and from supportive homes, and it seems incredible that they would have trouble with reading and spelling.

William's parents are intelligent and articulate and really supportive of him, but William was struggling at primary and intermediate school. Everyone told him not to worry, that he had a gift which was dyslexia, and that successful people are often dyslexic. One day he came home from school and told his parents, "I don't like my gift". William, like anyone, would rather be a good reader and writer than have a gift like that. Everyone was trying to make him feel better, but it is not enough. It is better to be able to read and write.

Ryan also comes from a very supportive and able family, and he is very talented himself. He laboured through primary and high school and got to university determined to do well, yet he struggled.

Esperance struggled at primary school, was frustrated, and doubted herself a lot according to her mother, but it was actually helpful for her when she was told she fitted the profile of dyslexia. She learned that she was not dumb, and that many famous people have had this profile. She said this made her feel better about it, that she didn't have to worry about it. This is the positive message about the profile of dyslexia. Yes, it is a label, but at the same time it recognises that you are not dumb, that you can get there: you can learn to read and write a whole lot better.

The nice thing about the stories of Ryan and William is that they were using the technology of the digital world we live in, including computers that can read books and lecture notes to them. At university Ryan was taking advantage of the services available, such as a note taker to sit with him in classes, and the recent innovation at university of having lectures video- and audio-recorded for him.

The video is very positive because you can see that dyslexia does not have to wear you down. We *can* teach students with dyslexia in more effective ways. We also have digital technology that can make learning easier so that these students can meet the challenges of education in today's world. The video shows that you can succeed even though life will be a bit tougher for you than for others.

An overview of the book

The message of the book is that we really need to get on top of this literacy problem. We talk around it, but we need a Department for the Prevention of Literacy Difficulties to identify early children who are at risk of dyslexia (and other reading problems), and we need to train specialist tutors who can help them and give them access to digital technology to make their classroom lives easier. Parents don't know what to do, and schools are struggling, yet we have a huge amount of research telling us that we can help these students. Now we need the political will to make it happen.

Following this brief introduction, Part One focuses on current knowledge of dyslexia. In Chapter 1 dyslexia is defined, and the difference between dyslexia and other types of reading difficulties are explained. Chapter 2 dispels myths associated with dyslexia.

Part Two presents two chapters on what it is like to live with dyslexia. Chapter 3 discusses the importance of the interactions between school and the family. The chapter presents data from two surveys of primary and secondary schools, which show that most schools have students with dyslexia, and that some schools are in a position to identify students with dyslexia, yet less than half are equipped to teach these students. We learn that dyslexics who have become successful have received considerable support from their parent/s. Chapter 4 is about dyslexia, self-esteem and behaviour. It explains that students with dyslexia often hide their difficulties and have to endure much criticism from their peers and lack of understanding from teachers. It explains how this affects their self-esteem and behaviour. We explain that there is much evidence that students with dyslexia need a support system early in their school careers.

Part Three examines the assessment of dyslexia. Chapter 5 describes the simple view of reading and writing and how dyslexia fits into this model. It explains how the student with dyslexia has average or better language comprehension but is poor at decoding and spelling. Chapter 6 is on screening for dyslexia. We outline a number of screening steps teachers can follow to determine whether a student is likely to have dyslexia. Assessment to gain official help, such as a reader–writer, usually requires a specialist report from an educational psychologist, but teachers can use various assessment measures to screen for possible dyslexia. The value of doing this is that it can give the teacher a clear direction as to what teaching tools are needed.

Part Four is all about how to help students with dyslexia. Chapter 7 focuses on teaching dyslexic students to read more effectively. Teaching reading is complex. It requires considerable teacher knowledge, commitment and the belief that the students will, in the end, learn to read. By the time children with dyslexia reach high school many have experienced years of less-than-positive reading experiences. This, combined with the increasing complexity of text, adds additional challenges, not only for the student but also for the teacher. This chapter presents an overview of the English language, because this knowledge is fundamental to teaching reading successfully. Lesson plans for teaching children to read are included in the Appendices.

Chapter 8 is about teaching how to spell effectively. Spelling is essential for writing. Of course a good speller may not be a good writer, because you have to have something interesting to say to be a good writer, but students with dyslexia often have interesting ideas. Their big problem is their spelling. The effect of having to put so much mental energy into spelling can range from annoying, such as the odd spelling mistake, to a complete turnoff because their written work is unreadable—and they know it. We explain lots of simple strategies that will get rid of simple mistakes, and the Appendices have more resources including a spelling programme of word lists, stretching over 22 weeks, to teach the basic Anglo-Saxon vowel patterns.

The focus of Chapter 9 is fluency. Fluency in the area of literacy is reading and writing with accuracy and speed. Many of us think that fluency is easily achieved—that you just have to force your eyes to read faster. One of us remembers, as a teacher, when our school purchased a speed-reading package that presented the text faster and faster to force our students to read more fluently. It was a disaster: it just made everyone's eyes ache from reading too quickly. We explain in this chapter that fluency comes with skill, and that we have to build up our reading and spelling skills so that they are effortless and automatic, such that we are able to process print without thinking, and this requires many hours and years of practice. In the chapter we explain the importance of fluency, especially for reading comprehension, and show how teachers can use effective strategies to increase fluency. Some ideas for developing fluency using Big Book reading are in the Appendices.

In Chapter 10 we explain how teachers can make their classroom dyslexia friendly. The chapter explains how to situate students with dyslexia so that they learn more effectively, and how to adjust classroom lessons to make them more successful. Creating a dyslexia-friendly classroom requires careful planning and preparation, but the benefits for the student with dyslexia—in fact all students—are significant. There are two video clips on this topic.

Part Five, in the form of Chapter 11, is the final word, in which we summarise the main messages of the book. Finally, the dices provide a wide variety of tools for assessing students with dyslexia and helping them to read and write.

The companion video

The companion video to this book (see www.nzcer.org.nz/nzcerpress/new-zealand-dyslexia-handbook), *Talking about Dyslexia*, has six segments, each about 5 minutes long. Three segments feature students with dyslexia: Esperance, who is in Year 6; William, who is in Year 8; and Ryan, who is completing a BSc, majoring in chemistry. One segment takes a brief look at a dyslexia-friendly classroom and school, and another focuses on 'What is dyslexia?' The titles of the segments are:

- Defining dyslexia
- William's story
- The dyslexia-friendly classroom

- Ryan's story
- The dyslexia-friendly school
- Esperance's story.

There are a number of ways of utilising the video clips. They could be viewed prior to reading the book, or individual segments could be viewed alongside the relevant chapters. The title segments and associated chapters are:

- Defining dyslexia   Chapter 1
- William's story   Chapters 2 & 3
- The dyslexia-friendly classroom   Chapter 10
- Ryan's story   Chapters 2 & 3
- The dyslexia-friendly school   Chapter 10
- Esperance's story   Chapters 2 & 3

Summary

Dyslexia is mysterious to many people, yet it becomes easy to understand once you have some information about it. We believe it is ignored by schools and the community because of a lack of understanding, and people have taken on ideas that are not backed by research. This book aims to address this. We aim to demystify dyslexia and show that there are many practical things classroom teachers can do about it.

The information in this book will complement the resource that is already available from the Ministry of Education's website, *About Dyslexia* (Ministry of Education, 2008). This book also complements another book we have written for the Tertiary Education Commission targeted at the adult level, called *Dyslexia Decoded*, which is available online with video clips, and also in print form (Dymock & Nicholson, 2013).

We have written this book and created the video clips with the aim of helping dyslexic students. This is an up-to-date resource. The authors are experienced university teachers and researchers with expertise in literacy. In putting the book and video clips together, we consulted with other university researchers, students with dyslexia, their parents, classroom teachers and principals. For years we have taught students with dyslexia to read and spell. We have listened to their stories (refer to the video clips featuring Ryan and William, who both attended the University of Waikato Children's Reading Centre). We have put together a comprehensive overview of current thinking about dyslexia and how to deal with it based on our reading of the literature and our experience working with many hundreds of struggling readers. The overall goal has been to produce a useful and practical resource for teachers and tutors working with school-aged pupils who have dyslexia.

PART ONE
GETTING TO KNOW DYSLEXIA

CHAPTER 1

What is dyslexia?

Dyslexia is an unfinished story

Dyslexia is an enigma. As we will explain in this chapter, dyslexia is a hugely researched area but the story of dyslexia is not yet complete. We know from neuroscience research that there is probably a genetic basis for dyslexia but we do not yet know the specifics and any practical implications of this research are still not yet available. There is not one story of dyslexia but many stories reflecting many opinions. In this book we argue that there are practical things that a teacher can do about dyslexia, things that we can do something about in the classroom. We know what the proximal indicators are, the things that stand out immediately, such as difficulties with reading and spelling. We know the sorts of instruction that will help overcome these difficulties. The distal indicators, that is, the genetic story, still has to be played out.

Prevalence

Estimates vary from 2 to 20 percent, but many agree that 10 percent of students have dyslexia and struggle with learning to read and write. Helping students with dyslexia is really urgent because the reality is that if a student falls behind in reading and writing they are unlikely to catch up with their peers without some form of intervention (Clay, 1987; Foorman, Francis, Shaywitz, Shaywitz, & Fletcher, 1997; Nicholson, 1997, 1999, 2000, 2003, 2008; Nicholson & Gallienne, 1995). In this chapter, we argue that students who have already received high-quality initial classroom instruction, yet are experiencing persistent difficulties in learning to read and spell, and who have particular difficulties in reading words phonologically, and who are developing normally in every other way, are likely to have dyslexia (Elbro, 1999; Goswami, 2008; Tunmer & Greaney, 2010).

Dyslexia: What is it?

How do you recognise a pupil with dyslexia when you see one? As noted in the Introduction to this book, the term *dyslexia* goes back more than 100 years and was originally used to describe a 14-year-old who seemed normal in every way, especially in language skills, but struggled with reading and spelling. This seemed surprising because most of us think it should be possible for everyone to learn to read and write, and it is even more surprising when someone who seems to have ability is unable to do this. The term *dyslexia* came to be used for students like this: those who have good language skills but still struggle to read and spell the words of their language. In the remainder of this chapter we will give a definition of dyslexia; explain that the New Zealand Ministry of Education and many researchers (Shaywitz, 2003; Shaywitz, Morris & Shaywitz, 2008; Torgesen, 2005; Wolf, 2007); write that we can help students with dyslexia learn to read; explain the simple view as a way to distinguish dyslexia from other reading difficulties; give a brief review of possible causes of dyslexia; explain that there are different opinions about dyslexia but conclude that dyslexia does exist; and that with help from this book teachers can do a great deal to reduce its negative effects on reading and writing.

Definitions

Tunmer and Greaney (2010) reviewed research on dyslexia and formulated a definition that has become well known and highly cited. They argue that students with dyslexia can be taught to read but they require longer and more intensive instruction. They define dyslexia in terms of four characteristics.
1. It is a persistent reading and writing difficulty
2. It happens to a normally developing student
3. It happens despite effective classroom instruction
4. It is because they have tremendous difficulty with phonological recoding, that is, in cracking the code of written language.

Can the teacher help students with dyslexia?

The NZ Ministry of Education (on its website) gives the reader links to resources to help with teaching students who have dyslexia: http://literacyonline.tki.org.nz/Literacy-Online/Student-needs/Learners-with-special-education-needs/Dyslexia

The Ministry website is very positive about the prognosis for dyslexia:

> Early identification followed by a systematic and sustained process of highly individualised, skilled teaching primarily focused on written language, with specialist support, is critical to enable learners to participate in the full range of social, academic, and other learning opportunities across all areas of the curriculum.

Indicators of dyslexia: proximal and distal

Distal indicators are those indicators that are not immediately obvious, such as something not right in neural processing, or genetic factors, or family background. *Proximal* indicators are those that are immediately obvious such as inability to read and spell. There has been a huge amount of work done in neuroscience looking for distal indicators that make it difficult for the dyslexic to learn to read and write, and much has been achieved but there is still not a consensus about these causes. The following section explains the two main points of view.

The genetic explanation of dyslexia

Milne (2014) reviewed a great deal of neuroscience and other research and concluded that dyslexia has a genetic cause. This genetic cause has been shown up in studies of identical twins where if one twin has reading difficulties it is likely that the other will as well. Genetic factors seem to result in neurological differences in wiring at birth. Evidence for this comes from post-mortem studies of brains of adults who were known to be dyslexic. Researchers found evidence of ectopias (or bundles of neurons that migrated to areas that normally do not have neurons) in the left side of the brain in areas responsible for language and reading. The ectopias were traced back to the sixth month of pregnancy.

Researchers have also found, using the technique of functional magnetic resonance imaging (fMRI), that there is less activation in the left hemisphere when the dyslexic person is reading and more activation in other areas, suggesting that the dyslexic person is compensating for lack of activation in the left hemisphere. This compensation process also happens when reading languages other than English.

Dyslexia can be a result of brain injury where the person was, before the injury, able to read but as a result of the injury lost ability to read. This is known as 'acquired dyslexia', as distinct from difficulty in learning in the first place, which is known as 'developmental dyslexia'. There are several kinds of acquired dyslexia:

1. One kind is **surface** dyslexia where the person can read words with regular spellings and can read non-words that have regular spellings but strikes trouble with exception words that have irregular spellings. People with surface dyslexia are sometimes called "Phoenician readers" because they are better at reading words phonologically.
2. Another kind of acquired dyslexia is **phonological** dyslexia where the person can read words that have irregular spellings and can read well-learned words but have trouble with unfamiliar, nonwords that have to be sounded out (but see the case study of Castles & Coltheart, 1996). People like this are sometimes called "Chinese readers" because they are better at reading exception words.

The reason for the two kinds of acquired dyslexia relates to the way our mind processes words and how a brain injury might affect this. In reading there are two routes that can be followed in reading words (Harley, 2010). One is the lexical route for well-learned words where we read them as sight words. The other is the sound route, or non-lexical route, where we use grapheme—phoneme correspondences to recode words according to their phonemes. A brain injury might knock out the lexical route and produce surface dyslexia, making it hard to read irregular or exception words. Or, a brain injury might knock out the non-lexical route and produce phonological dyslexia. This would make it difficult to read regularly spelled nonwords because the only way you can work these out is to sound them out.

Acquired dyslexia is different to developmental dyslexia. Developmental dyslexia, which is the focus of this book, occurs where there are no indications of brain injury and can be of the surface or the phonological kind. The reasons for developmental dyslexia are still being researched. Phonological developmental dyslexia is by far the most common kind of developmental dyslexia (Roberts, Christo & Shefelbine, 2011).

There does seem to be a genetic basis for dyslexia and it may be that the gene once had a positive role to play. It has created difficulties for the dyslexic reader but humans have been on earth for hundreds of thousands of years, long before the invention of literacy (which happened only about 5,000 years ago) and during this time the dyslexic gene might have had a positive contribution to make though we are not sure what. Some say it is a 'creative' gene but there is no clear evidence of that. The different wiring of those with dyslexia therefore might have had evolutionary value but it is only in recent times that it has come to cause difficulties for those with this gene who also need to have high levels of reading and spelling skill.

The limitations of neuroscience research

In contrast to the research reviewed by Milne (2014), Elliott and Grigorenko (2014) and other researchers (e.g., Goswami, 2012) suggest that the distal (neurological) causes of dyslexia are not yet known for sure. The argument is that we cannot compare dyslexic and non-dyslexic groups unless we have an agreed definition of dyslexia and this is not where we are at the moment.

They argue that many neuroscience studies are carried out without any consensus on how to define dyslexia. It seems that deciding who has dyslexia differs from one researcher to the next. This creates problems in that each study has its own way of defining dyslexia which may not be right. Elliott and Grigorenko (2014) gave an example of one recent neuroscience study that predicted future reading gains on the basis of brain activation during a reading task. They noted that to be classified as dyslexic you had to be in the bottom 25 percent of readers and in the normal range on an IQ test. The problem is that not all researchers agree IQ should be part of the definition of dyslexia. Elliott and Grigorenko argue that until we get an agreed definition of dyslexia it is hard to know whether neuroscience studies are telling us about dyslexia or about reading difficulties in general.

There is the possibility that difficulty with reading for the dyslexic pupil is because of prior poor reading experiences. Krafnik, Flowers, Luetje, Napoliello and Eden (2014), using fMRI technology, found that the brains of children with dyslexia (they also defined dyslexia as low in reading but average or better in IQ) were very similar to those of reading-matched but younger controls. They argued that differences in the dyslexic brain were not a cause of reading difficulties but a result of a long period of not reading very well and not reading enough to keep up with their peers. Elliott and Grigorenko (2014, p. 122) note:

> Currently we are unable to progress beyond a recognition that reading disability has a genetic component, or even an understanding of some possible specifics of those components, to a knowledge base capable of informing differential diagnosis and individualised forms of intervention.

Evidence from twin studies and many other studies indicate that dyslexia is heritable, that it has genetic and neurological origins. It is just that the expression of those genes depends on many other factors such as the environment in which the child is raised, the education they receive, and so on. Knowing that the distal cause of dyslexia is partly genetic is important but the difficulty for the teacher is in knowing how to deal with proximal causes, that is, how to diagnose and treat the student with dyslexia.

Stories of dyslexia: Adam

Adam seemed to fit the dyslexia profile perfectly: average or better listening (i.e. language) comprehension but considerable difficulty with the written code, as in oral reading, spelling, and writing. Adam was 8 years old at the time, from a school in a middle-class area, and he was from a very supportive family. He had been in some difficulties at school, mainly behavioural. He attended our university after-school reading programme for 2 years.

When he first came for after-school reading lessons we assessed his receptive vocabulary, that is, his knowledge of word meanings, we used the Peabody Picture Vocabulary Test (Dunn & Dunn, 2007) to do this. Each test page had four illustrations and the pupil had to point to the illustration that matched the test word, for example, "Look at these four illustrations and point to the fish". The test showed his vocabulary ability was at his age level but when we assessed his ability to decode aloud and his spelling it was a different story. He was reading words at a 6-year-old level and his spelling was the same. The results showed that Adam fitted the definition of dyslexia: he had average language skills for his age, but poor reading and spelling.

Adam came to reading lessons once a week after school, for 1 hour at a time. At first he was not keen to go to the lessons, but his mother bought him an ice-cream if he attended and this worked well. We trained university students to do the tutoring, and they followed a teaching plan designed to help Adam, which involved practising some phonics skills, doing some spelling, and doing some reading each week. At the end of the first year Adam was reading at an 8-year-old level and spelling at a 7-year-old level.

In the 2nd year of the programme Adam did even better. He was now 9 years old, and at the end of the 2nd year he was reading at nearly a 12-year-old level and spelling at an 8-year-old level, and his language comprehension score had jumped to a 10-year-old level. We didn't see Adam after that: his mother probably felt that the job was done and he didn't need lessons any longer. He was doing really well in reading and his spelling had improved. The lesson we learned was that you can teach students with dyslexia and they can make considerable progress. We can't be sure it was our teaching that led to the improvement. It might have been other teaching happening at school or at home. Whatever it was, Adam was now reading at a level that was right for his age. Adam fitted the category of dyslexia but his real difficulty may have been that he had not received appropriate instruction.

Should we even use the term "dyslexia"?: The debate

We will now review the arguments about using the term dyslexia. It is fair to say that the field is divided about this. Here are the arguments for and against.

1. Labels such as "dyslexia" are not helpful

One argument against the term "dyslexia" (Elliott, 2005, 2006; Elliott & Grigorenko, 2014) is that if you say someone is dyslexic it implies there is something wrong with them, that they have a "disability". This then could lead to lower expectations of them because teachers and parents may think they are not going to be able to meet the same challenges as their classmates. If you think your child or your students have dyslexia then you might also be drawn into trying programmes and ideas that say they will fix this disability, yet the programmes do not have scientific support (see Chapter 2 on misconceptions about dyslexia).

This is a concern but lower expectations and making bad decisions about how to treat dyslexia are really a problem of lack of information and possibly not knowing what to do to help. Also, we cannot assume that teachers and parents will give up on them because they have a label.

2. There is nothing special about dyslexia

Researchers are not agreed about whether dyslexia is a different condition. The argument is that it is a reading difficulty like any other reading difficulty. Most programmes to teach dyslexic students to read focus on phonics which is exactly the same reading instruction as given to other poor readers. If the instruction is the same then the reading difficulty must be the same (Elliott & Grigorenko, 2014).

However, this overlooks the distinction between the dyslexic reader who are most of the phonologic kind and the typical struggling reader. The simple view (that we explain in Chapter 5) tells us that the typical struggling reader needs help with both decoding (e.g., teach skills) and language (e.g., teach vocabulary and general knowledge). But we would not do this with a dyslexic student because, by definition, they already have average or better language knowledge. To treat them like a typical struggling reader, teaching them both phonics *and* language skills, means that you are teaching them some things they already know, and why do that?

3. Dyslexia is a way for middle class parents to get special treatment

Some researchers argue that the term dyslexia is favoured mainly by middle-class parents to get special treatment for their children, and that those with an economic advantage who manage to have their children diagnosed with dyslexia do this to get extra resources from the educational system. Riddell (2009) found that the boys and girls receiving instruction for dyslexia were mainly children of the middle classes.

However, this argument overlooks the fact that dyslexia can cut across all social classes, and that there are children from poor backgrounds who are average or above average in listening comprehension and fit the category of dyslexia. Their parents might not be able to afford to pay for a diagnosis, but that is no reason to limit the application of the term *dyslexia*: just because some social classes are better able to access the resources that are available. It should be possible for the government to ensure all social classes get access.

4. The definition of dyslexia excludes the poor

It is argued that definitions of dyslexia exclude pupils from poor homes on the grounds that their difficulties may be due to other factors, such as inadequate parenting. However, if we again use the simple view, children from poor homes would not be excluded. The simple view does not say that we must include only pupils from well-off homes. It applies to anyone.

5. Resources are diverted to one group who are privileged

Giving the label of dyslexia to a subgroup of children shifts the emphasis from supporting all students with reading/writing difficulties to an inequitable distribution of resources to those who have the label of dyslexia, leaving fewer resources to help other struggling readers. On the other hand, it would not necessarily lead to an imbalance of resources. It would be a more efficient use of resources in that the student in the dyslexia category does not need extra teaching of vocabulary and so on because although they may show some weaknesses in language their main difficulties are in decoding and spelling.

We do agree though that in terms of equity, it is not right that one subgroup should get special help and not others. We are saying only that it is helpful to have a label in terms of teaching so that we know what to focus on. The issue of equity is not a problem if the government provides funding that helps all struggling readers.

The reading and spelling miscues of students with dyslexia are similar to those of normally progressing but younger children

In reading and spelling, students with dyslexia make similar errors to those of younger but normally progressing children. The reason for most dyslexic children (the phonological type) seems due to the fact that they have so much trouble with phonological awareness and learning the alphabetic principle much more so than normally progressing children. As a result they do not learn so well how to decode words. This shows up in lower performance in reading non-words as in the Bryant Test of Basic Decoding Skills (see Chapters 6 and 7) and in their spelling.

Research on spelling shows this pattern of errors where the errors are similar to those of younger, normally developing children (Bourassa & Treiman, 2003; Cassar, Treiman, & Moats, 2005, 2006). It is the same for reading. An example is research by Thomson (1978) who compared two groups of 10-year-olds. One group was dyslexic and the other was made up of above-average readers of the same age.

What distinguished the two groups was that the dyslexic readers made more graphic and phonemic (decoding) errors compared with above average readers of the same age.

Thomson interpreted this to suggest that the dyslexic group were different to younger, developing readers who at the time were thought to make more semantic errors than decoding errors but Singleton (2005) pointed out, in a review of Thomson's study, that we now know that younger, beginning readers do make similar kinds of errors due to their reliance on guessing.

So it could be argued that dyslexic students with phonological processing difficulties are following the same track to reading and spelling as their peers but are way behind them due to their extreme difficulties with phonological recoding, difficulties that seem to strike them more than normally developing children. This is good news for the teacher in that it means quality instruction that combines authentic reading with teaching of phonics skills can help the student with dyslexia. They do not necessarily need something totally different from regular instruction. The challenge is to provide sufficient quality instruction for a long enough period of time, given that these students have persistent difficulties.

Dyslexia in the classroom

While the distal (underlying) indicators are being sorted out by neuroscientists, we can focus on the proximal indicators of dyslexia: the immediate factors that we *can* do something about and that are related to teaching. One way of tackling dyslexia is called the response to intervention approach. What this means is that the school provides three waves of instruction. The first is to start with quality classroom instruction (tier 1). Students who do not respond to this can be given small group instruction (tier 2). Students who do not respond to small group work are given one-to-one instruction (tier 3). An example of this is research by Vellutino et al. (1996). In their work they found that the percentage of below-average readers who were at risk of being categorised with dyslexia on initial assessment was reduced by two-thirds with quality classroom instruction that combined both reading practice and teaching of phonics skills. This was reduced again with follow-up small-group instruction of a similar kind, so that only a very small fraction of those who were initially at risk of dyslexia needed to receive one-to-one instruction, perhaps only 2 percent (Vellutino, Fletcher, Snowling & Scanlon, 2004).

A similar pattern of results was found in a further study, where classroom instruction as a result of professional development for teachers reduced the number of children at risk of dyslexia (Scanlon, Gelheizer, Vellutino, Schatschneider & Sweeney, 2008). This indicates that when students at risk of dyslexia are given quality classroom instruction that fits their needs the numbers reduce significantly (Gresham & Vellutino, 2010; Vellutino et al., 2004). In these studies the instruction had an emphasis on phonological decoding skills combined with reading practice, which has a stronger effect than other approaches (Ehri, Nunes, Stahl, & Willows, 2001; Hattie, 2009; Tse & Nicholson, 2014).

Calfee (1983, 1984) argued in articles titled 'The mind of the dyslexic' and 'The mind of the reading teacher' that many pupils in our schools with dyslexia are in classrooms where teachers are unable to teach them adequately because in their training they did not learn skills for teaching students with dyslexia. This suggests that we could provide more effective teaching in the classroom but it requires much more professional development for teachers in how to teach students with dyslexia.

Dyslexia at home

Students with dyslexia often come from very supportive and literate homes where they are surrounded by books. So books at home and reading books to children at home cannot be the main reason for their lack of success in literacy. Parents can identify tell-tale signs very early on that a child is at risk of dyslexia, especially if they seem like a regularly developing pupil but are close to starting school with little or no alphabet knowledge or phonemic awareness. Parents *can* take action. Much research suggests that teaching phonemic awareness at home and the letter-sounds of the alphabet before children start school can reduce the risk of them falling behind in reading. In this new digital age, families can also source apps that build alphabet and phonemic knowledge (e.g., Profs' Phonics, which is a nice little app to teach letter sounds).

Parents can still read books to their children but we suggest include attention to letters and sounds when reading. A suggestion is to read books that directly promote phonemic awareness and letter knowledge such as books with rhymes and alliteration and ABC books. For example: Quentin Blake's ABC or Dr Seuss's ABC. Phonemic awareness books include: *Each Peach Pear Plum*, *Hairy Maclary from Donaldson's Dairy*, *The Cat in the Hat*, *Don't Forget the Bacon*, and *How Many Trucks can a Tow Truck Tow*?

Summary

This chapter has given a brief coverage of the many theories and debates about dyslexia in the literature. As the reader will have noticed, dyslexia is much debated and still not resolved—it is a real enigma. The focus has been on proximal indicators of dyslexia, on finding a practical way of sorting out the student with dyslexia from other pupils with reading difficulties and providing instruction that is targeted to their specific needs—decoding and spelling. In the near future, neuroscientists may well be able to tell us the distal (genetic/neurological) indicators that are linked to the wiring of the dyslexic brain. We are not there yet.

In the meantime the proximal (immediate) indicators of dyslexia are that these students experience persistent reading and spelling difficulties, despite classroom instruction provided by experienced teachers, even though they are developing normally like other pupils, and for the reason that they have serious difficulties in phonologically decoding what they read. In terms of teaching, these students need intensive teaching and for a longer period of time than for other students. When classroom teachers and specialist tutors implement effective instructional skills (which this book provides) they can reduce dramatically the numbers of dyslexic students struggling with literacy.

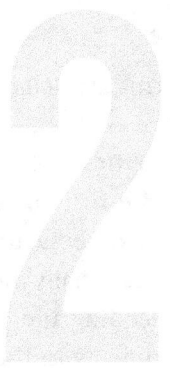

CHAPTER 2

Misconceptions about dyslexia

Introduction

There are many ideas and theories about dyslexia and there are many programmes that claim they can help dyslexia. Some of the programmes say they are backed by neuroscience but there is not much support for these claims (Coltheart & McArthur, 2012). In this chapter we review some of the most popular ideas and summarise the research on them. We suggest that some beliefs about dyslexia are not backed by research and some programmes are not supported either.

We accept that there are individual cases where improvements for the better seem to happen as a result of using these programmes but we think this is due to a novelty effect of doing something new. It is also the case that if you unconsciously think the treatment is working or that it might work, it sometimes does—this is called the placebo effect. It does not mean the programme is effective. Instead it says something about how powerful the mind can be. All the ideas we look at in the chapter are popular in some places and there are those who sincerely believe in these ideas but we argue they are misconceptions in that there is no clear research to back them up.

Dyslexia is related to intelligence

In the past dyslexia was defined in terms of intelligence. A significant gap (e.g., a 2-year gap) between intelligence level and reading and spelling level was seen as indicating dyslexia. Many researchers now argue that this is not a good way to define dyslexia. The problems these students have with reading and spelling are not related to their intelligence (Stanovich, 1996). Instead, other factors are better predictors of success in reading (Gresham & Vellutino, 2010), especially those most related to the act of reading and writing, such as phonological decoding and spelling difficulties.

The thing is, high-IQ and low-IQ students are different in many ways, but the cause of their reading/spelling problems is not different: it is due to problems with phonological recoding; that is, reading and spelling words according to their syllables and phonemes. If a student is articulate and seems average in every way, we expect them to be able to read and spell, so it comes as a surprise when they do not. This makes it even clearer that intelligence is irrelevant to literacy difficulties, because these difficulties cut across every social class and the whole range of intelligence.

Dyslexic students have different learning styles

Many of us think that we learn better if the material to be learned uses a learning style that we like. For example, some people think they learn better if the material is in a visual format, such as pictures or graphs, while others think they learn better when they listen, others when the learning is hands-on, etc. The idea of learning styles is widespread in the general workplace and in education. For example, a recent survey found that 82 percent of graduate teacher trainees about to enter secondary school teaching thought that teaching pupils in their preferred learning style could improve their learning (Howard-Jones, 2011). However, there is little evidence to support this idea, mainly because many of the learning styles ideas have not been tested, and the ones that have showed no effects (Pashler, McDaniel, Rohrer, & Bjork, 2008). Corballis (2011, p. 224) wrote about learning styles in this way:

> Of course those with good verbal skills may well gravitate towards careers in journalism, law, or (heaven help them) academia, while those with good visual skills may well become artists, architects, or professional tennis players. What is unclear from the literature is whether the learning of any accomplishment, be it algebra, art, or critical writing, can be tuned to people's different aptitudes. The evidence remains stubbornly negative.

Dyslexia is a male problem

It is often the case that most of the students who receive tuition for literacy difficulties are males. In the Reading Recovery programme more than three out of four pupils are males, but could this be a result of a selection bias, so that males are more likely to be picked out as having difficulties? It seems that boys are seen as being worse behaved than girls, and this leads schools to attend more to their reading problems. Girls appear better behaved and they don't get the same attention in school, even though many of them struggle to read. Researchers have found that when you assess both boys and girls there are similar numbers who have literacy difficulties and that boys are seen by teachers to have more behaviour problems, which may indirectly result in more boys being selected for special tuition (Prochnow, Tunmer, Chapman, & Greaney, 2001; Shaywitz et al., 2008).

Dyslexia takes time to show itself

In fact it doesn't really take much time to show itself. If students starting school are assessed and they fit the profile of dyslexia, then this is an indicator of future difficulties. Children who start school low on these skills do not progress very well (Nicholson, 2003). Pre-reading skills of alphabet knowledge and phonemic awareness (sometimes called literate cultural capital) are strong predictors of later literacy progress (Judge, 2013). We can know very early on if a pupil is at risk for dyslexia, we do not have to wait for them to fail.

Dyslexia will go away over time

It is tempting to think that reading difficulties are developmental, and that for most pupils they will go away as children mature and they continue through school, but this is not the case. It seems that reading difficulties will persist without some kind of intervention, and the gap between good and poor readers will not close over time, and may even increase (Judge, 2013; Shaywitz et al., 2008).

Dyslexia is a visual processing problem

Students with dyslexia often reverse letters and words; for example, they read *on* as *no*, or *b* as *d*, *dog* as *god*, and so on, but researchers have found that the tendency to reverse words and letters is no greater in dyslexics than in other poor readers. It is a result of not being able to read—not a cause of it. If you do not read very well, you will not have the letters in a word stored securely in memory, so that when you see another word that has a similar look to it you are likely to get confused. This is what beginning readers and spellers do as well, so it is not peculiar to dyslexia. The research on this topic indicates that focusing on visual training does not help, and that the best strategy is to teach directly phonological recoding skills; that is, how to decode words (Vellutino et al., 2004).

Dyslexia is a balance problem

Some researchers have found a positive result for balance exercises to help dyslexia, but the results have been strongly criticised (see the critique by Bishop, 2007, and a letter to the editor by Reynolds and Nicolson, 2008). Programmes that offer these exercises cost a lot of money but do not have any strong evidence to support them (Stephenson & Wheldall, 2008).

Dyslexia is helped with coloured overlays

Pupils sometimes say that the words jump around on the page, or that the words flicker or are fuzzy. Some people have argued that this is overcome by the use of coloured paper, or coloured overlays, or coloured lenses, but there is little research to support this claim. Northway (2003) found only small gains in rate of reading, and these may have been due to a placebo effect. Other studies have found no effect for coloured paper, overlays or lenses (Handler & Fierson, 2010; McIntosh & Ritchie, 2012; Palomo-Alvarez & Puell, 2013; Ritchie, Della Salla, & McIntosh, 2011; Van Kuyk, 1995).

Evidence for a placebo effect is a randomised controlled trial in New Zealand, in which 24 children aged 8–12 years practised using coloured overlays they selected themselves and also overlays they did not select themselves but which were selected for them (these were placebo overlays). The results after 6 weeks showed no significant difference between the two kinds of overlays. More than half the children selected overlays that matched their favourite colour. The most frequently selected overlay colour was blue (Van Kuyk, 1995).

Summary

There are many different ideas about how to overcome dyslexia. How do you choose which one to go with? The best way is to look at the research. The ideas covered in this chapter do not have enough research support to warrant investing in them. Learning styles, balance exercises, coloured overlays—the list goes on. Those who have tried these ideas may have found them helpful but it might have been a placebo effect, that is, the effect of thinking that something might be helping you. The mind is very powerful and this probably explains why some with dyslexia have gained from these treatments. It is just that the scientific research does not show they are effective. A suggestion, if you are interested in a programme that is supposed to be a cure for dyslexia, is to read as much as you can about the research, and to read independent research, not just the studies that are on the website of those who want you to buy their product.

PART TWO
LIVING WITH DYSLEXIA

CHAPTER 3

Dyslexia, family and the school

Introduction

Imagine how a parent feels if, despite doing all the right things—such as reading books to them every night and buying them lots of children's books—their child struggles to learn to read when they start school? It comes as a total surprise in that there is no apparent reason why this should happen. The child seems normal in every respect, they have a wide vocabulary, they have a really good understanding of things explained to them or read to them, and yet they find it hard to get into reading and writing. As time goes on at school the young reader starts to lose confidence and thinks they never will learn to read and write. They may get grumpy, not want to go to school, and avoid reading and writing altogether. This is often the profile of a student with dyslexia. In this chapter we start to look at how parents and teachers can approach this problem. Detailed discussion and advice about specific interventions are provided in Part Four.

Are schools able to deal with dyslexia?

If a child fits the profile of dyslexia, we recommend that their parents talk with the school about it, and if possible see an educational psychologist to get an opinion. If parents are unable to afford an assessment like this, then choosing the right school will be really important. Parents should find out as much as they can about the school. Does it recognise dyslexia? Are there teachers at the school with specialist training, or with a particular interest in dyslexia or reading difficulties? How does the school keep parents informed of the help that is offered? What type of training have they had? Does the school operate a pull-out programme (i.e. students pulled out of their normal classroom for specialist tuition), or is the additional help classroom based? Are extra-curricular activities offered? In other words, what systems are in place to help students with dyslexia?

It may be that the school doesn't have systems in place, and this is understandable in that schools have only recently become aware of the nature of dyslexia. Dyslexia is officially recognised by the New Zealand Government, and the Ministry of Education have a working definition (see Chapter 1) and have published a brochure on dyslexia, *About Dyslexia*, which is easily downloadable from the internet,[1] but many schools may still not be totally up to speed with dyslexia.

We base this claim on the results of a survey we emailed to school staff in December 2011 and December 2012 to gauge their understanding of dyslexia and how they assist this group of students. We sent the survey to more than 500 schools in the Waikato and Auckland areas and received responses from 42 schools in the first survey and 26 in the second survey. The responses were from a range of school staff—from teacher aides, to teachers, to school leaders, including principals. The survey only tapped into a small number of schools, but given that there is very little information from schools in the literature, we thought it worth sharing the results. (We do understand that schools must receive many survey requests: one principal wrote, "I didn't respond to your survey. I receive so many surveys that I simply can't respond to them all".)

Table 3.1: School survey on dyslexia

Survey question	Percentage responding yes	
	2011	2012
Do you have students with dyslexia in your school?	98	96
Can your school identify students with dyslexia?	64	65
Do you have procedures to deal with dyslexia?	62	54
Is your school equipped to teach students with dyslexia?	40	12

---

1 literacyonline.tki.org.nz/content/download/15836/.../About+Dyslexia.pdf

Our interpretation is that the results were fairly similar for 2011 and 2012, except for the question about being equipped to teach students with dyslexia: in the 2012 survey 12 percent of respondents felt they were equipped to do this, whereas in 2011, 40 percent felt they were equipped. The *overall* results for the two surveys were that 97 percent of the respondents said their school had students with dyslexia, 64 percent said they could identify such students, 59 percent said their school had procedures to deal with dyslexia, and 29 percent felt equipped to deal with dyslexia. It was interesting that nearly all respondents said their schools had students with dyslexia and that most of the respondents felt they could identify them and had procedures to help them, but the result of most interest to us was that less than one in three respondents felt equipped to deal with dyslexia. The results of this small survey suggest to us that staff in schools are still a long way from feeling comfortable about their ability to help students with dyslexia.

Dyslexia and stress at school

Stress factors in the classroom

While there is a fun factor associated with school (e.g., playing or hanging out with friends, school trips), we also know that school is associated with stress (Thomson, 2004). Many high school students become stressed when they sit tests, when assignment deadlines are near, when preparing and presenting speeches, and when NCEA exams are looming. Students from the age of 5 can also experience school-associated stress. Stress is simply a part of life. However, school-related stress is exacerbated when students experience reading and writing difficulties, or if a student is dyslexic. One reason for dyslexia-related stress at school is that it takes a student with dyslexia longer to process and produce text.

Stress is part of everyday life, but it becomes threatening when it is "pervasive and invasive, when it affects too many areas of our lives and when we have neither the strategies nor the energy to cope with it" (Thomson, 2004, p. 3). If each day at school you encounter reading material you should be able to read yet are unable to, or you are required to write answers, stories, or articles and you struggle to spell, it is likely that stress levels will increase and become "pervasive and invasive". Even if a student with dyslexia can decode the text, they do so without fluency. When decoding and encoding are required, dyslexic students are always behind. Dyslexia simply robs people of time. There is a fine line between stress that inhibits or debilitates, and stress that enables individuals to achieve: "If stress levels become intolerably high, many dyslexic children develop their own inappropriate strategies, becoming disruptive, aggressive, withdrawn or school phobic" (Thomson, 2004, p. 4).

Personal experiences of dyslexia: Henry Winkler

The American actor Henry Winkler (the Fonz from the 1974–1984 television series *Happy Days*) knows about school and stress. He experienced considerable challenges at school due to dyslexia. Winkler has shared some of his not-so-positive school experiences with writer Lin Oliver, and together they have co-authored a series of children's books based on an 'underachieving' boy, Hank Zipzer. The 17 books have become a *New York Times* best-selling series.

The series stars a child who has learning disabilities (or dyslexia) yet is "really smart and fun".[a] Winkler and Oliver wanted to "speak to kids and to let them know that inside each one of them they have a special and unique contribution to make". As Winkler put it, "No matter what obstacle might be in your way there is a way around it. There is a way to beat the obstacle and continue to your dream."[b]

The titles in the Hank Zipzer series by Henry Winkler and Lin Oliver include:
- *Help! Somebody Get Me Out of Fourth Grade*
- *Summer School!*
- *What Genius Thought Up That? The Night I Flunked My Field Trip*
- *I Got a "D" in Salami*
- *Niagara Falls, or Does It?*

Many plots in these stories link directly to negative school experiences, such as *I Got a "D" in Salami* and *Niagara Falls, or Does It?* Both of these books demonstrate that school was not stress-free for the main character, Hank, which draws on Winkler's own school experiences. Hank is bright, intelligent and enjoys having fun. One thing Hank does dread is school. Is this a typical characteristic of children with dyslexia?

The following is from the book description for *I Got a "D" in Salami* (Winkler & Oliver, 2003a):

It's report card day—the most dreaded day in Hank's school year. And when Hank gets his grades, they're his worst nightmare come true: a D in spelling, a D in reading, a D in math. After school, Hank and his friends go to his mom's deli. His mom is on the prowl—she knows a report card day when she sees one. Hank tries to stall her, but she's going for his backpack. He's cornered. Hank hands the report card off to his friend Frankie, who gives it to his friend Ashley, who gives it to Robert, who puts it into a meat grinder! Hank watches as his Ds are ground into a big salami, and this particular salami is being made for a very important client. How will Hank get out of this one?

Here is the book description for *Niagara Falls, or Does It?* (Winkler & Oliver, 2003b):

For Hank, fourth grade [Year 5] does not start out on the right foot. First of all, he gets called to the principal's office on the very first day of school. Then the first assignment his teacher gives him is to write five paragraphs on "What You Did This Summer". Hank is terrified—writing one good sentence is hard for him, so how in the world is he going to write five whole paragraphs? Hank comes up with a plan: instead of writing what he did on vacation, he'll show what he did. But when Hank's "living essay" becomes a living disaster, he finds himself in detention. Strangely enough, however, detention ends up becoming a turning point in his life.[c]

[a] http://www.hankzipzer.com/video.html.
[b] http://www.hankzipzer.com/video.html.
[c] Both quotations are from http://www.hankzipzer.com/books.html

Eissa (2010) assessed 56 12–18-year-olds, who were divided into two groups: poor readers ($n=35$) and typical readers ($n=21$). There was no significant difference in chronological age, IQ or socioeconomic status between the two groups. Eissa found that most of the poor readers were male, and that dyslexia "caused them to feel different" (p. 19). Dyslexia had a negative impact, either "quite a lot" or "very much" on their self-esteem. Most of the poor readers felt their difficulties with reading and writing had had a negative impact on their relationships with their peers. Some had been bullied or teased. Two comments reported in the study were, "The best moments in school were the breaks" and "the only thing I enjoyed was playing with my classmates" (p. 19). Students also reported feeling uncomfortable in school (e.g., "I felt I was the most stupid child in class") and feeling optimistic about the future: they will be "better off" once they leave school.

Providing the kind of help and support for dyslexic students so that they do not feel embarrassed is not easy. A New Zealand interview study (Rowan, 2010) of four New Zealand university students with dyslexia asked them about their high school experiences. One participant reported that "they made me go to an English tutor" and "they treat you like a kid" (p. 75). Another student said the high school support was "embarrassing and humiliating" (p. 75). The same student felt embarrassed the way the teacher singled her out in front of her peers. The student said, "I'd be sitting in class and the teacher would go like talking about something and then just turn around and look at me and say 'did you understand that' in front of everyone!" (p. 76). Rowan (2010) reported that the relationships the four participants had with their friends, teachers and parents/family "played an important part in their attitude to learning and acceptance of their learning struggles" (p. 76).

Acknowledging dyslexia is the first step

The first challenge facing the teacher is to come to an opinion about dyslexia. There are stereotypes of the pupil with dyslexia that teachers needs to be aware of. For example, Riddick (1996) reported an interview with a teacher in the UK who was sceptical about dyslexia (pp. 94–95):

> **Interviewer:** Have you done any specialist training in the area of dyslexia?
> **Teacher:** Oh God that. No, no I haven't [pulls a face].
> **Interviewer:** Why did you pull a face when I asked you that?
> **Teacher:** Well … I mean, it's one of those things that has been conjured up by 'pushy parents' for their thick or lazy children: quite often both.
> **Interviewer:** What exactly do you know about dyslexia?
> **Teacher:** Well, basically they can't read or write. It's supposed to be about problems

with communication isn't it? Generally it's children who are either too lazy or haven't got the brains and their parents can't hack it.

Later in the interview:

Interviewer: If you haven't any training in the field of dyslexia do you think really that you should be making judgements about it?

Teacher: Yeah, it's a gut feeling you know, when you have been teaching as long as I have you get to know which kids have problems and which kids are pulling the wool over your eyes. (Riddick, 1996, pp. 94–95)

The interview shows that there are sceptical opinions about dyslexia, but we believe there is a category of struggling reader who fits the dyslexia profile. As we have noted, the Ministry of Education also recognises dyslexia, and this is another good reason for teachers not to dismiss it and to think about how the classroom programme could be adapted to help a student with dyslexia.

What would a dyslexia-friendly classroom look like? It would be one where the teacher feels they want to help students with dyslexia. That is a great start. The next step is to find out what dyslexia is: to have a working definition that will enable the teacher to assess and identify the pupil with dyslexia and distinguish them from other pupils who have literacy difficulties. In Chapter 1 we did this (gave a definition), and in Chapter 6 we give ideas on what to assess.

The next step is to build some teaching strategies that will help. In Chapters 7 and 8 we give some ideas for doing this in reading and spelling. A final step is to set up communication with the parents of a student with dyslexia so that they are both on the same page and working with each other. We do this in Chapter 10, where we talk in detail about how to make the classroom a dyslexia-friendly place to be. (Refer also to 'The dyslexia friendly school' in the companion video *Talking about Dyslexia* (see http://www.nzcer.org.nz/nzcerpress/new-zealand-dyslexia-handbook).

Dyslexia and the home

For the classroom teacher it is really important to make a connection with the home so that the teacher and the student's parents are working together—are on the same page. In one of the video clips that accompany this book there is an interview with William's mother (William is one of the case studies; see 'William's story'). William's mother was reluctant to contact the school about his lack of reading and spelling progress because she did not want to "be a middle-class parent breathing down the teacher's neck." The teacher can break down this reluctance by getting in touch with the home.

Establishing good relationships between the child, parents/care-givers and the school is important for all children, but especially for children with dyslexia. Establishing positive relationships involves considerable knowledge and understanding, at many levels. What knowledge and understanding are needed? Both teachers/schools and parents need to have:
- an understanding of dyslexia
- an understanding of the impact of dyslexia on the child's learning (reading/spelling)
- an understanding of the impact of dyslexia on the child's self-esteem and feelings of self-worth
- the ability to communicate with the child
- the ability to communicate with each other.

The pupil with dyslexia will benefit if they have:
- an understanding of dyslexia
- an understanding of how dyslexia affects reading and spelling skills.

The number one goal for parents and teachers is to preserve the child's self-esteem (Shaywitz, 2003). Students with dyslexia are typically bright children, and it comes as a surprise—and often a shock—that they have reading and writing difficulties. Students with dyslexia struggle with reading and writing, and as a result do not usually get their school work completed. This makes it seem as if they are not working hard enough and that they need to do more, when in fact they are really working hard but their reading and writing difficulties are like major traffic bottlenecks that stop them from doing what their classmates can do. If we keep thinking they are not working hard enough and keep giving that kind of feedback, then they will start to doubt that they can succeed (Shaywitz, 2003).

Shaywitz (2003, p. 309) talks about the "extraordinary perseverance" the student with dyslexia must put into their reading and writing, and we can acknowledge this by supporting them, praising them and giving them more time. Shaywitz notes that "all dyslexics who have become successful by any account share in common the unfailing love and support of their parent(s), or occasionally, a teacher or a spouse" (p. 309).

Conclusion

In this chapter we have discussed dyslexia in relation to the classroom and the parents, and have indicated the importance of positive and effective connections among teachers, pupils, their parents, and the school. Schools and teachers may not feel fully equipped to deal with dyslexia, and this is probably because it has only recently become officially recognised. Dyslexia, when it occurs, takes us by surprise. It usually happens to students who seem to have everything going for them, and if we lived in a society that did not have reading and writing they would seem normal in every way. The key to giving them the best possible help is for teachers, parents and the pupils themselves to work together in a positive and supportive way.

CHAPTER 4

Dyslexia, self-esteem and behaviour

What is life like for the student with dyslexia? In this chapter we will review research showing that students with dyslexia often hide their difficulties and have to endure much criticism from their peers and lack of understanding from teachers. We will also look at how this affects their self-concept, self-esteem and behaviour.

Real-life examples

One way to gain insight into the self-esteem of students with dyslexia is to read personal accounts. Robert Frank wrote a book on the experience of dyslexia. In the book he reflects on his childhood as a dyslexic: "As a child, I was called dumb. I was called lazy. And that was just by some of my teachers. You can imagine the names that the kids in the school yard added to that list" (Frank & Livingston, 2002, p. 1).

Another personal account is that of actor Henry Winkler, referred to in Chapter 3. In a talk given at Benchmark School, a highly rated school for bright students with dyslexia in Pennsylvania, Winkler shared some of his childhood experiences:

I was told I was stupid and I believed it. My father could speak 11 languages and do math in his head. He was confounded that I was in the bottom three per cent academically in this country. He always pushed me to concentrate, because if I concentrated I would get it. If I sat at my desk long enough, I would get it. (A conversation with Henry Winkler, 2010, p. 3)

Brenda Millward had dyslexia and wrote in a book chapter that she accepted she was "slow and lazy" at school (Millward, 2004, p. 139). She had difficulty enunciating the sound of the letter *r* and this became the butt of jokes. As a result, she avoided talking at school.

In tthis book's companion video (http://www.nzcer.org.nz/nzcerpress/new-zealand-dyslexia-handbook) there is a profile of William, an intermediate-age student with dyslexia (see 'William's story'). An interesting aspect of the interview relating to self-esteem is that he was told in school he had not written enough and had to write another page. To William this request from the teacher seemed like asking him to do the impossible. When William had to answer written questions, he asked his friends to help him by reading them out loud to him because of his decoding difficulties. He didn't want to make a fuss. He tried not to burden just one or two of his classmates, and so he asked a number of them to help. William's mother's response to his situation was, "What a way to have to live your life." Other indications of low self-esteem from his parents were that he was anxious about school; for example, he didn't sleep well and he had the habit of tugging on his lip.

Self-concept and self-esteem

Self-concept is the "individual's view of himself or herself" (p. 116) and our "ideas about our attributes and abilities" (Sternberg & Williams, 2010, p. 388); or, as Ridsdale (2004, p. 250) puts it, "our sense of self". The study of self-concept is complex and beyond the scope of this book, so we have used Shavelson and Bolus's (1982) model of self-concept, a model that has received empirical support, to help readers understand this term. Their hierarchical model of self-concept is shown in Figure 4.1.

Shavelson and Bolus's model shows general self-concept at the top of the hierarchy. At level two self-concept is split into academic and non-academic. At the third level these two sections are split again: academic into subject areas and non-academic into emotional, physical and social self-concept. This splitting is called *differentiation*. Self-concept becomes differentiated as we acquire more skills and learn more about what we can and cannot do. As a result, we may have high self-concept in some areas, such as sport, but low self-concept in other areas, such as academic tasks. Or we may have high self-concept in maths but low self-concept in English.

Figure 4.1: The structure of self-concept

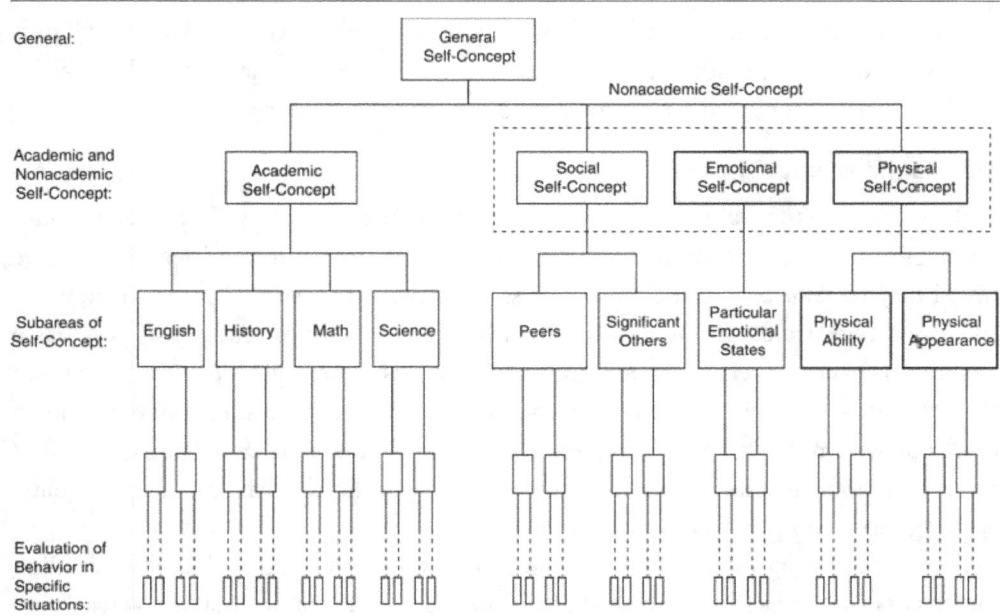

Source: Shavelson & Bolus, 1982, p. 7.

Self-esteem is related to self-concept. Self-esteem is the ideas one has about one's attributes and abilities and "the value that an individual places on himself or herself" (Sternberg & Williams, 2010, p. 116). Brooks (cited in Ridsdale, 2004, p. 260) defines self-esteem as "based upon the feelings and thoughts that individuals possess about their sense of competence and worth". Self-concept is what you *know* about yourself, but self-esteem is what you *feel* about yourself. For example, you may know that your parents and your friends think you are terrific, but you may not feel the same as they do. The way you feel about yourself is your self-esteem.

Self-concept can be mapped onto self-esteem so that self-esteem can be separated into different areas, including academic and non-academic, and subsets of these two areas, such as reading, writing and maths. If teachers hope to raise the self-esteem of their students with dyslexia—or of all students—in essence "they are hoping to change the way someone thinks and feels both about what they can and can't do and also about how valuable they are" (Ridsdale, 2004, p. 263).

Literacy instruction is obviously crucial for improving the reading and writing skills of students with dyslexia, but we also need to find ways of teaching that help to raise their self-esteem.

Strategies for raising self esteem

Effective literacy instruction in itself can help to raise self-esteem because it will give positive feedback to the student who is improving. They will see they are reading harder book material and writing or composing longer and more interesting work.

Metacognitive strategies

Metacognition is the ability to think about your own thinking. Good readers use metacognitive strategies. Good readers know how they think and learn and have the ability to take control of the process. Students with dyslexia may not develop metacognitive strategies. One reason for this is that a lack of reading success has a negative impact on their ability to develop these kinds of strategies. We can teach them metacognitive strategies when we are teaching them to read and spell. For example, in this book we emphasise explaining the reasons for what we teach and the logic behind the instruction, such as explaining how the history of the English language has made spelling more complex than it used to be.

Another metacognitive strategy is to get the student to ask themselves if the reading material is making sense. If they ask this question, and it is not making sense, then they stop and figure out what is going wrong. It means taking control of literacy rather than letting it control you. For example, in word reading, a positive metacognitive strategy is, when you make a mistake, you try to fix it or get help, whereas a negative metacognitive strategy is to give up. In the stories in the companion video clips to this book (http://www.nzcer.org.nz/nzcerpress/new-zealand-dyslexia-handbook) William, Ryan and Esperance all had positive metacognitive strategies. They were not letting dyslexia control them.

Taking the ego out of reading and writing

The effective instructor explains to the student with dyslexia that it is all about getting the task understood and done, and not about getting frustrated or upset. Encourage them to be cool and not get upset if they do not get it the first time. If the student is struggling to get on top of a skill, explain that they should not feel good or bad about it: it is a skill to be learned, and it *will* happen.

Teachers should make use of praise. It is amazing how little we praise students. We are not good at giving praise even though we all like it when we get it (Nicholson, 2014). Students with dyslexia especially need praise because they already feel so bad about themselves. Research suggests that behaviour-specific praise that tells the reader or speller what they have accomplished is the most rewarding for the student with dyslexia. Less effective praise is general praise, like "Good boy". Bennett's (2009) study of exemplary reading tutors found that tutors use both types of praise: praise with no feedback (e.g., "Good girl"), and praise with specific feedback (e.g., "Good boy. I like the way you broke that word into syllables" (p. 29), although the research indicates that praise involving feedback about the behaviour being praised is better.

Peer group support is important. In this book's companion video the part that covers 'The dyslexia friendly classroom' explains that students in a dyslexia-friendly classroom support one another. This might be very simple, such as a classmate explaining instructions or reading out a piece of text for the student with dyslexia. The video explains how this can be reciprocal: William supported some students in writing vocabulary because he had such a wide vocabulary, and others supported William in decoding text. Other forms of support might be peer tutoring or cross-age tutoring.

Increasing a sense of self-efficacy

Self-efficacy "is an individual's belief in his or her potential to succeed in a particular situation" (Ridsdale, 2004, p. 271). Whereas self-esteem is how you feel about your abilities, self-efficacy is your sense of how capable you are. The teacher needs to challenge any feelings of learned helplessness; that is, when a dyslexic student thinks they cannot do something because they have failed in the past. The teacher should work steadily towards building a sense of competence in the student that they *can* do things, and this might be step-by-step, which involves breaking the task down so that success comes with mastering one small chunk at a time; for example, learning how to read three-letter regular words, then learning to spell them, and so on, providing challenges that bring success.

Panagos and Dubois (1999) found that dyslexic adolescents' self-efficacy has a limiting influence on their career choices (see also Ridsdale, 2004). A low sense of self-efficacy can lead to denying that they are able to do something when in reality they can. Bandura's (1993) seminal research reports that if the task is considered too difficult, we do not try hard or persist. Failing, again, only reinforces the belief that the task cannot be completed successfully. Changing these long-held beliefs takes time and much more than comments such as 'Well done' or 'Good' or what Ridsdale (2004) refers to as "warm fuzzies" (p. 271). Ridsdale (2004) reports that even when some children with dyslexia first experience success in literacy they are quite aversive. Their belief that they will not succeed has been "rattled" and, again, this places them in a position of risk. The risk this time is that they have been in a position of learned helplessness—they have been onlookers. Now, with the literacy skills they have developed, they are "in the race" (Ridsdale, 2004, p. 271).

Behavioural issues

Hiding difficulties

Brenda Millward (2004) wrote that she hid her difficulty by avoiding talking. Children's author Patricia Polacco (1998) tried to hide from fellow classmates so that she wasn't taunted during interval. Each morning she would go to the bathroom just before interval, and instead of returning to the classroom she would hide under the stairwell. Patricia felt safe there from the cruel comments of her classmates.

Shaywitz (2003) wrote about a university student who described dyslexia as "the beast, and unknown predator that silently stalks him, constantly disrupting his life" (p. 4). Another student, Charlotte, studying law, hid her difficulties for fear her lecturers would question her ability. Shaywitz wrote that "with all the stereotypical views of dyslexia, she reasoned her professors would have second thoughts about her abilities" (p. 5), so she felt caught: "If I take extra time, they'll all think I don't deserve my grade and that I'm really not so smart. If I don't take extra time, I'll never finish" (Shaywitz, 2003, p. 5).

Consider the challenge of hiding your reading and writing difficulties throughout your school years, when much of school time is spent reading and/or writing. The following examples of classroom timetables in primary and secondary school (see Tables 4.1 and 4.2) illustrate the large amount of time the student spends reading and writing in any one school day. We estimate that more than 3 hours is spent engaged in reading-related activities and 2 hours in writing.

Table 4.1: Timetable for a typical Year 4–6 school day

Time	Topic	Reading	Writing
9.00	Day begins Roll, homework, news	No	No
9.15	Language (i.e. reading, writing, spelling)	Yes	Yes
10.30	**Interval**		
10.50	Maths	Yes	Minimal
12.00	PE	No	No
12.30	**Lunch**		
1.15	Unit studies (social studies, science, health)	Yes	Yes
2.15	Other activities such as library visits, assembly, music, art, drama,	Possibly	
3.00	**School day ends**		

Table 4.2: Timetable for a typical high school day (Years 9–10)

Time	Topic	Reading	Writing
8.45	Form class	Possibly if announcements or notices are in written form	No
9.00	English	Yes	Yes
10.00	Maths	Yes	Yes
	Break		
11.30	PE	No	No
12.30	**Lunch**		
1.15	Social studies, science, or languages	Yes	Yes
2.15	Other activities such as assembly, music, art, drama,	Possibly	Possibly
3.00	**Day ends**		

The effects of criticism

Whether criticism is intentional or accidental it can have a negative effect on all of us. Dale Carnegie, who wrote classic books on self-help, suggested that we should never give anyone criticism, and it is good advice, yet it happens all the time. We discussed earlier in the chapter that Robert Frank (Frank & Livingston, 2002, p. 1) was called "dumb" and "lazy" by some of his teachers, and he left us to imagine what his peers called him. Children's author Patricia Polacco was called "dummy" by her classmates. They asked her why she was "so dumb" as she stumbled over words she was asked to read by her teacher (Polacco, 1998). Henry Winkler was told he was "stupid", and he believed it (A conversation with Henry Winkler, 2010, p. 3), and his parents called him "dummer Hund," which is German for "dumb dog". Scottish racing driver Jackie Stewart is also dyslexic, and he said this:

> You will never understand what it feels like to be dyslexic. No matter how long you have worked in this area, no matter if your own children are dyslexic, you will never understand what it feels to be humiliated your entire childhood and taught every day to believe that you will never succeed at anything. (Wolf, 2007, pp. 165–66)

The following high school students' comments help to illustrate that school life is not what it may seem on the outside (National Institute of Child and Human Development, 2000b, n.p.):

> Teachers, I don't think sometimes mean to make fun of people who can't read well. And it really gets tough.

> Because school is tough. And everyone is trying to look for a way to fit in. And anyone who doesn't at all, really gets ripped to pieces.

> Some people don't want to be laughed at.

> And they just start to decide that maybe the human race isn't such a great thing after all.

Dyslexics may react in different ways to the failure they are experiencing. Edwards (1994) explains that a student with dyslexia who has an introverted or shy personality tends to remain quiet and stay in the background. In contrast, a student with a more extroverted personality might react in the opposite way by attracting attention, becoming aggressive, being argumentative or the troublemaker. Their main objective would be to distract attention from their real frustration/problem—their difficulty with reading and writing. One high school student with dyslexia commented, "I remember a lot of times I just tried to always take the back desk. Keep my head down, keep my hand down, and keep my mouth shut" (National Institute of Child and Human Development, 2000b, n.p.).

The power of knowledge

Shaywitz (2003) argues that once a child understands why they are experiencing difficulty learning to read and spell, they are "greatly relieved" (p. 310), which has a positive impact on their self-image and how they view themselves (note William's and his mother's comments in 'William's story', in this book's companion video, *Talking about Dyslexia*, (see www.nzcer.org.nz/nzcerpress/new-zealand-dyslexia-handbook) when they were informed that William has dyslexia). Parents and teachers play a significant role in building self-image. Shaywitz (2003) writes that the student should be told that their difficulty is shared by many other people, ordinary people as well as extraordinary people (e.g., the actors Henry Winkler and Tom Cruise, rocket scientist Kettler Griswold, entrepreneur Sir Richard Branson). Reassure the student with dyslexia throughout their primary and high school years that their difficulty is not due to lack of intelligence.

Shaywitz (2003, pp. 310–311) also argues that parents and teachers should talk to their child about dyslexia so that they have a good understanding of what is known about dyslexia and to assure them they are not on their own. In addition, parents and teachers should explain to the child that:
- he/she will learn to read
- learning to read and spell is much more challenging for someone with dyslexia
- dyslexia affects many different people from all walks of life
- dyslexia can run in families, but even though one family member has dyslexia it does not mean other family members will.

Esperance (see 'Esperance's story', *Talking about Dyslexia*) was diagnosed with dyslexia in primary school. After she was told she had dyslexia she found learning about famous dyslexics helpful. Teachers and parents can share stories with their children about others who have dyslexia. Henry Winkler did not understand why he struggled throughout his schooling until his son Jed was diagnosed with dyslexia. At the age of 31 years he realised that he had "something with a name" and that he wasn't stupid or lazy, and that the reason he was not living up to his potential was that he had dyslexia.

Over time, Winkler developed strategies for dealing with his reading and writing difficulties. One strategy was to remain positive: "If a negative thought popped into my head, I'd say, 'Sorry, no time for this now,' and replace it with something positive" (Wiseley, 2010). Winkler, once the "king of negative thoughts" (A conversation with Henry Winkler, 2010, p. 3) shared an important message with staff and parents at Benchmark School, Pennsylvania, a school for bright students with dyslexia (Wiseley, 2010)

> You're the advocate for your children. Their job is to dig up their gift and give it to the world, and your job is to support them in that. I used to hate my dyslexia—I wanted

to carve it out of my brain with a spoon or something. But now I realize that maybe I wouldn't be here if I didn't have it. Maybe I'm lucky to have it. And maybe these kids are too.

The difficulty is that many students with dyslexia, like Winkler, just don't understand why they are experiencing great difficulty learning to read and spell. Knowing why they are experiencing reading and spelling difficulty, and that they can learn provided they receive the right type of intervention, can make a significant difference (see 'William's story' and 'Esperance's story' in the companion video *Talking about Dyslexia*).

PART THREE
ASSESSING DYSLEXIA

CHAPTER 5

Dyslexia and the simple view of reading and writing

Introduction

Many of the ideas in this book are based on the simple view of reading and writing (Dymock & Nicholson, 2013; Gough, 1993, 1996; Gough, Hoover, & Peterson, 1996; Gough & Tunmer, 1986; Nicholson, 2005) because it is a useful way of understanding the needs of struggling readers. We have assessed hundreds of children coming to our after-school reading programmes over the years using assessments based on the simple view of reading and writing, and our data show that poor readers are not all the same, which is what the simple view says.

This seems like important practical knowledge for a teacher to have. The simple view of reading and writing separates students into four kinds who have to be taught differently. If we take reading, the categories are:

- the reader—average or better in decoding,[2] listening comprehension, and reading comprehension

---

2 There are many ways to define decoding but in this chapter we refer to it as oral reading accuracy.

- dyslexic reader—has average or better listening comprehension but below average decoding and below average reading comprehension
- language comprehension difficulties—can decode but cannot understand
- mixed problems—difficulties with decoding and also poor listening comprehension

The categories also apply to writing. The students who fit the dyslexia profile are usually really good at language but are poor decoders and spellers. They are a definite category no matter what you want to call them. As pointed out in Chapter 1, when you use reading/spelling age-matched controls, the reading and spelling difficulties of these children with dyslexia are similar to those of younger children. So their problems are not special: they basically can't decode or spell, and usually respond well to phonics, but they are definitely good at language, whereas the other two categories of poor reader are not. Our experience is that the ones in the dyslexia category usually do succeed and come up to average—but they argue with us all the way because they are good at talking! We don't give them instruction in language skills (e.g., vocabulary, general knowledge) because they are already good at that.

Since we use this model of literacy for assessing and teaching pupils who fit the profile of dyslexia, it is best if we now explain it in detail.

The simple view of reading

The simple view of reading is that reading comprehension can be explained as having two basic parts:
- decoding skill, or word recognition, as in the ability to read real words or made-up words accurately out of context
- listening comprehension, as measured by the ability to understand a text if it is read aloud.

Where does dyslexia fit into the simple view of reading? As we noted above, the model says there are four kinds of reader (see Figure 5.1).

Figure 5.1: The simple view of reading

	Poor listening	**Good listening**
Good decoding	**Language comprehension issues**—Is average or better in decoding but below average in listening comprehension and in reading comprehension possibly because not enough vocabulary or general knowledge, or a language impairment of some kind	**The reader**—Is average or better in decoding, in listening comprehension, and in reading comprehension
Poor decoding	**Mixed problems**—Is below average in decoding, in listening comprehension, and in reading comprehension	**Dyslexic reader**—Is below average in decoding yet has average or better listening comprehension but also is below average in reading comprehension

These different kinds of reader tend to have characteristic reading miscues (see Figure 5.2).

Figure 5.2: Kinds of reading miscues for the four kinds of reader

Text: The king and queen lived in a castle	Student reads:
Dyslexic reader	"The king and queen lived in a cottage. Well that's strange, I would have thought they lived in something better than that."
Language comprehension issues	"The king and queen lived in a castle. What's a castle?"
Mixed problems	"The kong and quin lifted in a cuddle. Weird, eh?"
The reader	"The king and queen lived in a castle. I wonder if it was damp?"

1. **The reader** will read accurately and understand what they read. For example, if the story starts off with "The king and queen lived in a castle" the student will read exactly those words and show understanding, such as thinking, "I wonder if the castle was damp? How long ago was it?"
2. **The dyslexic reader** will misread the words, but because of their good listening skills they might make a meaningful guess at the meaning. For example, "The king and queen lived in a cottage. Well, that's strange. I would have thought they lived in something better than that but that's their choice."

3. **Language comprehension issues** will have trouble understanding the text even if it is read aloud to them. This might happen to an immigrant pupil learning English as a new language (ESL), or to a student whose parents have English as a second language, or a student with a language impairment. This student will read the words correctly but will not know what they mean; for example, "The king and queen lived in a castle. What's a castle? What's a queen?"
4. **Mixed problems** will not know how to decode many words and will not understand very well what they read either, even if the material is read aloud to them, for example, "The king and queen lived in a -----. Well, I'm not sure where they lived." They experience the "double whammy" because they are below average in decoding as well as language comprehension.

As can be seen in Figure 5.1, when it comes to reading, the pupil with dyslexia has average or better language understanding but struggles with decoding. They are better off than the mixed problems poor reader in that their language skills are fine and they would understand the text if it was read aloud to them. They mainly need help from the teacher to build their decoding skills. In contrast, the mixed problems poor reader needs help with both decoding and language.

The simple view of writing

According to the simple view of writing (Juel, 1988, 1994; Juel, Griffith, & Gough, 1986), writing can be explained as having two parts:
- spelling, as in the ability to spell words correctly
- ideas, as in the ability to generate interesting ideas to write about.

According to the model, there are four kinds of writer (see Figure 5.3).

Figure 5.3: The simple view of writing: the four kinds of writer

	Poor ideas	Good ideas
Good spelling	Good spelling but has writing difficulties due to lack of ideas	The writer—has good spelling and ideas
Poor spelling	Typical struggling writer—has poor spelling and ideas	Dyslexic writer—has good ideas but poor spelling

1. **The writer** has strong spelling and good ideas and will write accurately and interestingly; for example, "It was a fine day, the sun was alive and shining, and the birds were singing a boetiful melody."
2. **The weak spelling but good ideas writer** may be able to get good ideas down, though the poor spelling will make the writing seem low in quality; for example,

"It wsa a fie doght, the sun was alain and shaesit, and the brisd were sig a boo midy."
3. **The poor ideas but strong spelling writer** will spell many words correctly but their ideas do not make sense—they do not communicate effectively; for example, "It was day, the sun, and the birds."
4. **The mixed problems struggling writer**, is poor in spelling and low in ideas, and is classified as a common-or-garden variety writer to indicate that this is the most common kind of writing difficulty; for example, "It wsa doght, the sun, and the brisd".
5. **The student with dyslexia** (as in the Type 2 writer above) has good ideas but will probably not be able to write them down due to their difficulties with spelling. They are likely to write slowly and make mistakes. They are better off than the mixed problems poor writer in that they do have good ideas. They need to improve their spelling and the other mechanics of writing, including punctuation and even handwriting.

A causal model of how we learn to read and write

Research by Juel, Griffith, and Gough (1986) found support for a model of learning to read and write that followed a sequence where certain skills contributed to the acquisition of the next skills needed for reading and writing (see also Juel, 1994).

Figure 5.4a: A model of reading acquisition (based on Juel, Griffith, and Gough, 1986)

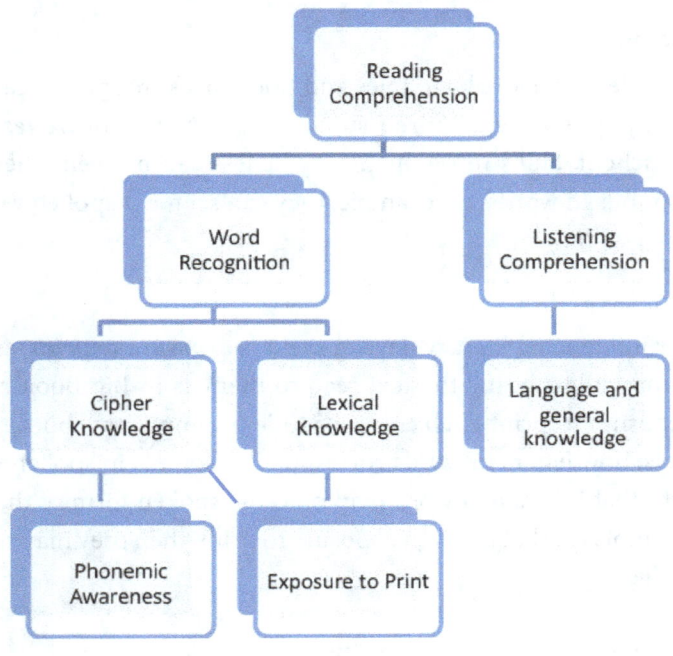

Figure 5.4b: A model of writing acquisition (based on Juel, Griffith, & Gough, 1986)

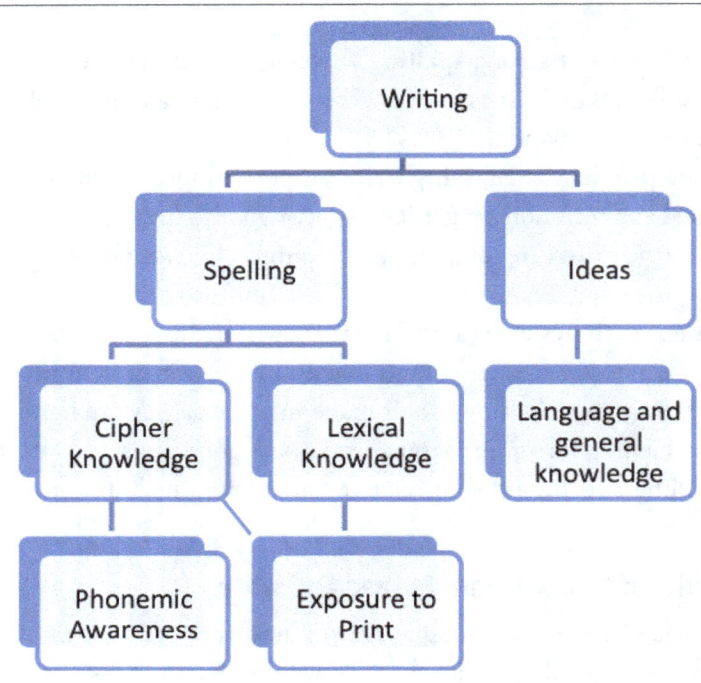

The components of the model are explained in detail below.

Prerequisites for reading and writing

Phonemic awareness

The mediating role of personal variables and home background appear to influence whether or not pupils have acquired sufficient *phonemic awareness* skills when they first start school. Skills in phonemic awareness can be seen when pupils have awareness of sounds in words; for example, they can segment spoken words like *teeth* into phonemes: *t-ee-th*.

Exposure to print

The next factor influencing literacy development is *exposure to print*, as when pupils look at the print while hearing the text read to them as in Big Book reading in the classroom. Exposure to print enables pupils to learn implicitly about the alphabetic principle; that is, how letters in words correspond to sounds in spoken words. If they have the insight that letters in a word map onto the spoken form of the word, and if they can get examples of that through exposure to print, then they may start to acquire cipher knowledge.

Language and general knowledge

This reflects the language experiences you have had as part of growing up. It also seems to depend on the ability you were born with and perhaps dialect (Seidenberg, 2013).

Cipher knowledge

Cipher knowledge is knowledge of the alphabetic principle. This principle says that letters in words correspond to phonemes in spoken words. But the cipher, though crucial, is still not enough because many words we read and spell will not have regular letter–sound correspondences. To read and write these irregular patterns we need lexical knowledge.

Lexical knowledge

The cipher will help pupils to read regularly spelled words like *cat* or *fan*, but not irregulars like *have* (the child may say 'hayve'), or *great* (the child may say 'greet') or steak (the child may say 'steek'). Many very frequently occurring words are irregular in some way, such as *was*, *come* and *what*. Pupils will misspell them using cipher spellings, such as *woz*, *kum* and *wot*.

As pupils continue to read on their own, they will learn these unusual spelling cases. While reading they will come across the irregular spellings and will make a mental note of their unusual spelling patterns. The model calls this **lexical knowledge**.

Reading

According to the model, if the pupil has cipher knowledge and lexical knowledge, then these skills will enable reading and writing—though they will take different paths. Let's look at reading first.

Word recognition

The child who acquires cipher knowledge first is equipped to acquire lexical knowledge. With both, the child will acquire skills of **word recognition**. Skill in word recognition enables the pupil to read both regular and irregular words.

Listening comprehension

Listening comprehension (i.e. the ability to understand spoken language) is the basis for reading comprehension. If listening comprehension is good, then the pupil will be able to understand the text if it is read aloud. The simple view says that reading comprehension requires adequate listening comprehension as well as adequate decoding (or word recognition).

Reading comprehension

This is the ability to read with understanding. The model requires the pupil to have good word recognition and listening comprehension in order to read with understanding.

Writing

Spelling

Cipher and lexical knowledge will have an impact on ***spelling***. The cipher speller can produce invented spellings but needs lexical knowledge as well in order to spell correctly the irregular patterns (like *come* instead of spelling it as *cum*), or the ambivalent forms, where one sound can be spelled in two or more different ways (e.g., whether to spell *green* as *grean*, *grene* or *green*). So the cipher speller must learn exceptions to the rules as well. The term *lexical knowledge* refers to the exceptions.

Ideas

According to the model, the writer needs ***ideas*** as well as spelling. The model keeps spelling and ideas separate from each other because some poor writers can spell but they lack ideas, while other poor writers have ideas but they can't get them onto the page because all their mental energy is going into spelling words correctly. If a poor speller with good ideas is asked to explain ideas aloud, then he or she will be able to give a much better impression of the extent of their ideas.

The simple view says that writing involves skill in spelling and the ability to generate ideas. Writing does not happen in the absence of ideas, and it doesn't happen in the absence of spelling. It needs both. Writing is the ability to express ideas with good spelling. Spelling includes punctuation (and handwriting in the absence of computers), but writing also involves generating ideas—writing with your own "voice".

Summary

The chapter started by explaining that the best way to assess dyslexia is to use the simple view of reading and writing. The simple view shows the difference between dyslexia and other kinds of reading difficulties. We also showed a path model of literacy acquisition that indicates what elements we can assess to find out the reasons for particular issues that show up during assessments. For example, we know that in the initial stages of learning to read and write, phonemic awareness is an issue for struggling readers and writers. This skill helps with spelling and with decoding words. In the later stages of reading and writing other aspects of the model are more important, such as vocabulary and the generation of ideas. The simple view gives a road map of what to assess. In Chapter 6 we apply the ideas discussed in this chapter to look at ways of assessing students for dyslexia.

CHAPTER 6

Screening for dyslexia

Introduction

How do you screen for dyslexia? An educational psychologist would be the most expert person to do this but the classroom teacher can do some preliminary assessment. We argue that the best way to do this is to make use of the simple view of reading and writing, which we introduced in Chapter 5. According to this model, the best way to screen for dyslexia is to check that the pupil has below-average decoding, above average listening comprehension, and below-average reading comprehension.

The model says that if listening comprehension is appropriate for their age and yet their reading comprehension is below age-appropriate level then the key difficulty for the dyslexic pupil is decoding. The chapter will explain in more detail how to assess their decoding skills.

How can the teacher use the model in the classroom?

The simple view says that by carrying out some simple assessments you can place all the pupils in your class according to their reading status. There will be four types of reader:

1. The reader—average or better in decoding, listening comprehension, and reading comprehension
2. Dyslexia (decoding difficulties)—below average in decoding, average or better in listening comprehension, below average in reading comprehension
3. Language comprehension difficulties—average or better in decoding, below average in listening comprehension, and below average in reading comprehension
4. Mixed problems—below average in all three areas.

The value of the simple view is that it helps the teacher to decide what action to take to improve the reading and writing of their class. A simple **action plan for reading** would be:

Figure 6.1: Action plans for teaching

	Listening comprehension	
Decoding skills	Below average	Average or better
Average or better	Type 3—language problems: Lesson plans will focus on building vocabulary and general knowledge through lots of reading mileage such as Big Book reading, discussion of vocabulary in the Big Books, general discussion of text meaning	Type 1—the Reader: build advanced comprehension skills through reading mileage, building vocabulary, and teaching comprehension strategies
Below average	Type 4—Mixed problems: Take a combined approach that focuses on building both decoding skills and language knowledge using Big Books to teach decoding skills and new vocabulary meanings	Type 2—Dyslexia: Build decoding skills through phonemic awareness and phonics strategies but in combination with reading mileage using Big Books to show how phonics patterns apply in context

To illustrate, Figure 6.2 is Ms Nickleby's classroom. This year she has quite a few pupils who are having reading difficulties. She has assessed all her pupils and placed them into the categories that fit the model. To do this, she found out which stanine each pupil was in. Many standardised tests place pupils in stanines from 1–9, with 1 being the lowest level, 5 is average and 9 is the highest level. She has also colour coded the test results according to ability levels.

As you can see, in her class she has some pupils with no reading difficulties but she also has quite a few pupils who are either in the dyslexia category or who are typical struggling readers. She has one pupil in the "language comprehension problems" category. The chapter will explain how you can assess these three areas for each pupil in your class.

For example, 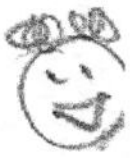 (indicated with a ***) fits the dyslexia category in that she is below average in oral reading accuracy as measured by a standardised word reading test (stanine 3), average in listening (stanine 5), and below average in reading comprehension (stanine 3). In support of the low word reading test score she also has a low decoding score on the Bryant Test of Basic Decoding Skills (BTBDS). The chapter will explain how to administer this test and will also give references to standardised tests so that the teacher can assess word reading accuracy (which is a surrogate for decoding skills), listening comprehension, and reading comprehension.

Figure 6.2: Ms Nickleby's classroom—showing the different kinds of reading status for her pupils

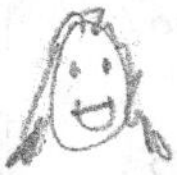

Ms Nickleby's class—Year 4

| Above average (6-9) | Average (5) | Below Average (4) | Well Below (1-3) |

Class Roll	Reading Difficulty Status	Word Reading Accuracy	Listening Comprehension	Reading Comprehension	Bryant Basic Decoding Skills
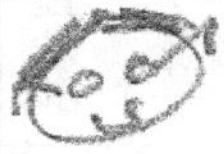	Mixed	2	4	2	15
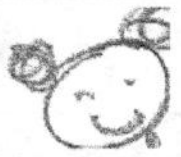	Mixed	3	3	2	18
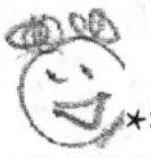 ***	**Dyslexic**	3	5	3	12
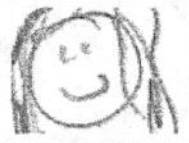	Reader	6	7	6	47
	Dyslexic	3	5	3	16
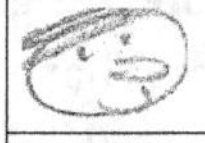	Reader	6	9	6	40
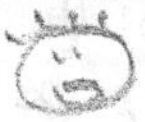	Reader	8	8	7	43

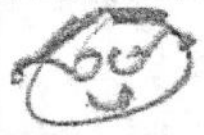

	Reader	6	5	5	33
	Reader	6	5	5	36
	Reader	8	6	6	49
	Reader	8	9	9	42
	Reader	8	5	5	47
	Reader	8	6	5	44
	Dyslexic	3	5	3	18
	Dyslexic	2	8	2	9
	Language	7	3	4	39
	Dyslexic	2	5	3	12
	Mixed	1	4	2	15
	Mixed	3	1	2	20
	Mixed	4	4	3	27
	Mixed	4	4	3	28
	Mixed	1	4	1	10
	Mixed	4	1	2	25

Steps to take to decide if a student has dyslexia

The steps are summarised in Figure 6.3 and described in more detail in the following text. However, in brief, the first step is to find out if the student really does have reading comprehension difficulties. Sometimes students think they are worse than they really are. If there are no difficulties, then the student does not have dyslexia and the assessment can stop. The second step is to check if the student has average or better language (listening) comprehension. If there are no difficulties with listening comprehension, and yet the student has difficulty with reading comprehension, then the cause must be with decoding, so move to the third step, to find out what aspects of decoding are giving difficulty.

Figure 6.3: Three steps in screening for dyslexia

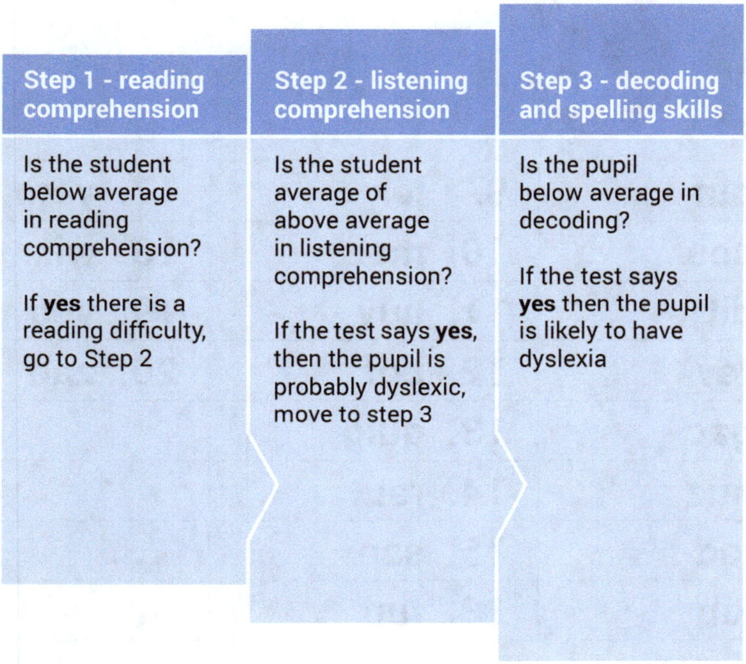

Step 1 - reading comprehension	Step 2 - listening comprehension	Step 3 - decoding and spelling skills
Is the student below average in reading comprehension? If **yes** there is a reading difficulty, go to Step 2	Is the student average of above average in listening comprehension? If the test says **yes**, then the pupil is probably dyslexic, move to step 3	Is the pupil below average in decoding? If the test says **yes** then the pupil is likely to have dyslexia

Diagnosing Decoding Skills—The Alien Words Test

Pupils with dyslexia struggle with decoding. The Bryant Test of Basic Decoding Skills (BTBDS) (Bryant, 1975; Nicholson, 2005) assesses decoding skills of different types. We explain to the students that this is an "alien words" assessment. This test presents non-words that follow the letter–sound rules of English. The tutor explains to the pupil that these are not real words: they are the words spoken by aliens from another planet, and they have to sound them out. The student reads one list after the other but testing usually stops if they make 10 consecutive mistakes. A complete copy of the test is in Appendix 1B. In this chapter, we will discuss different sections of the test to show how they link to phonics skills.

Instructions: "The words in this list are alien words. They are words from an alien language. Can you read them?"

Figure 6.4: A check on ability to read simple three-letter (CVC) words

Alien Words, Section 1

CVC (consonant-vowel-consonant) words. List includes single consonants and short vowel sounds.

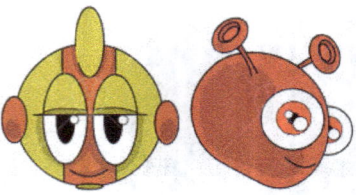

1. buf	9. lek	17. vom
2. cos	10. maz	18. wix
3. dit	11. nuv	19. yeg
4. fev	12. pof	20. zad
5. gac	13. quig	
6. huz	14. rel	
7. jod	15. san	
8. kib	16. tup	

The 20 alien words in section 1 assess ability to read simple three-letter words where there is a CVC pattern (consonant-vowel-consonant).

Problem—Unable to read CVC words

Each mistake can reveal something about the pupil's knowledge of letter sounds. For example, the student reads as follows:

Test word	Pupil's response
lek	look
san	sun
yeg	yog

These miscues indicate the pupil does not have a firm understanding of the short vowel sounds. He is able to read the consonant first and last letters but has difficulty with the vowel sounds in the middle of each word. He is also trying to think of real words. We tell the students that the words are "alien", not from this planet, so if the pupil does give a real word then explain again that the words are alien.

Solutions:

- Teach how to decode phonically regular VC and CVC words taken from their Big Books and other readers that have these patterns, e.g., *The King's Birthday* has the VC word "it" and the CVC words "cut" and "sat". The book *Watchdog Who Wouldn't* includes words such as "dog", "box", "Dad", "leg", "ran".
- Use dot-to-dot phonics where you draw three dots for the CVC word and ask the pupil to think of the first sound, the letter to go with the sound, and so on, e.g.,

•	•	•
s	a	t

- Teach short vowel sounds—see lesson plan in Appendix 6
- Teach short vowel phonograms—see Appendix 6
- Make phonics strips—see Appendix 4(c)

Figure 6.5: A check on ability to read words that have the silent e rule (CVCe)

Alien Words, Section 2

Silent e words with CVCe patterns

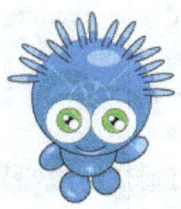

21. fute
22. yode
23. bime
24. nepe
25. cabe

The five words in Section 2 assess the student's ability to read words that follow the silent *e* rule. The rule is that the *e* at the end of the word does not have a sound but is a marker to tell the reader that the vowel before it says its name.

Note: This is not the only thing that the silent *e* does—it also is used in English spelling when words end in a "v" as in "give" and "love". In these situations it does not indicate that the preceding vowel has its long sound. The early printers used the *e* this way because they did not like words to end in *v*. It has other uses as well—we will look at this in the chapter on spelling. In this test, however, none of the items end in *v* so the silent *e* rule will apply.

Problem—Applying the "silent *e*" principle

How do you know if the pupil lacks understanding of the silent e principle? For example, the student reads as follows:

Test word	Pupil's response
fute	futtee
yode	yoddee
bime	bymee
phune	funny

In the above example, the pupil's difficulties with the silent *e* show up because she is pronouncing the *e* at the end of the word. She does not realise the *e* is a marker to tell her to pronounce the preceding vowel by its name.

Solutions:

- Teach how to decode some silent *e* words from their Big Books and other readers that have these patterns, e.g., *The King's Birthday* has the words "name", "cake", and "surprise". Before you read the book to the class, write these words on the whiteboard and read out the sounds of the letters slowly, pointing to each letter as you say the sounds so that students can see the decoding process at work: n-a-me, c-a-ke, s-ur-p-r-i-se
- Use dot-to-dot phonics where you draw three dots for the CVC(e) word and ask the class to think of the first sound, the letter to go with the sound, and so on , and to add the silent *e*, as in:

•	•	•
c	a	ke

- See the lesson on silent *e* in Appendix 6
- Teach short vowel phonograms in Appendix 6
- Make phonics strips using lists in Appendix 4(c).

Figure 6.6: A check on consonant digraphs

Alien Words, Section 3

Consonant Digraphs ch, sh, wh, th and long vowel sounds. List includes end-of-word long vowel sounds (cho, shi, whe) and silent *e* rule for long vowel sounds (thade, phune).

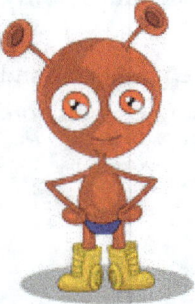

| 26. phune |
| 27. cho |
| 28. shi |
| 29. whe |
| 30. thade |

This check assesses whether the pupil knows consonant digraphs: *ph*, *ch*, *sh*, *th*, and *wh*. The *h* is a marker to indicate that these letters do not have their regular sound but a new sound.

Problem—Does not know the sounds of ph, ch, sh, wh, th

For example, the student reads as follows:

Test word	Pupil's response
phune	poon
cho	koe
shi	sie
whe	we
thade	tade

In the above example, the pupil's difficulties with consonant digraphs show up because she is using the regular sound for each letter. She does not realise the *h* is a marker to tell her to pronounce these letters differently.

Solutions:
- Select several consonant digraph words from their Big Books and other readers that have these patterns, e.g., in *The King's Birthday* there are the words "bir<u>th</u>" and "bir<u>th</u>day". Add some other words like "<u>th</u>in", "w<u>hich</u>", "<u>ch</u>ip" and "<u>sh</u>op". Write the words on the whiteboard and point to each letter as you say the sounds slowly, as in: b-ir-th-d-ay.
- Use dot-to-dot phonics where you draw three dots for the three phonemes and ask the class to think of the first sound, the letter to go with the sound, and so on, until you have all the phonemes for the word, as in:

b	ir	th
•	•	•

Figure 6.7: A check on consonant blends and vowel digraphs

Alien Words, Section 4

Initial consonant blends (e.g., st, pl, fl, sm, bl, cl, tr, sp, gr), r-affected vowels (er, ar, or), and vowel digraphs (one sound: aw, ew, ee, ai, oy, oa; 2-sound: oo)

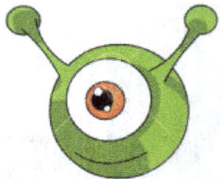

31. staw	36. cleef
32. plew	37. troob
33. fler	38. spail
34. smar	39. groy
35. blor	40. groaf

The alien words list will indicate if the pupil knows how to say consonant blends like *sp*, *gr*, *tr*, and so on. It also checks if they know the sounds of vowel digraphs like *ai*, *oy*, and so on.

Problem - Unable to read consonant blends or vowel digraphs

For example, the student reads as follows:

Test word	Pupil's response
staw	stoy
plew	ploe
blor	blar

This indicates that the consonant blends are known but not the r-affected vowels (e.g., the "or" in "blor" and the vowel digraphs (e.g., the "aw" in "staw").

Solutions:

- If consonant blends are a problem, use the lesson plan in Appendix 3(c)
- Use the vowel digraphs lesson plan in Appendix 3E and Appendix 6.
- Teach how to decode similar patterns from their Big Books and other readers, e.g., *The King's Birthday* has the "oo" pattern in "cooks" and "looked", the "or" pattern as in "ordered" and "doors", and the "ar" pattern as in "garden". Before you read the book to the class, write these words on the whiteboard and read out the sounds of the letters slowly, pointing to each letter or digraph as you say the sounds so that students can see the decoding process at work: c-oo-k-s, l-oo-k-ed, or-d-er-ed, d-oor-s.
- Use dot-to-dot phonics where you draw three dots for the CVVCC word and ask the class to think of the first sound, the letter to go with the sound, and so on, and to add the silent *e*, as in:

c	oo	k	s
•	•	•	•

- Make phonics strips using lists in Appendix 6.

Figure 6.8: A check on multi-syllable words

Alien Words, Section 5

*Multi-syllable words: some words have English **prefixes** (<u>de</u>fev, <u>pre</u>fute, <u>un</u>cabeness, <u>ex</u>yoded); some have English **suffixes** (gac<u>tion</u>, uncabe<u>ness</u>, exyo<u>ded</u>, sanwix<u>able</u>, bufkibb<u>er</u>, vomaz<u>ful</u>); some have neither (cosnuv, relhime)*

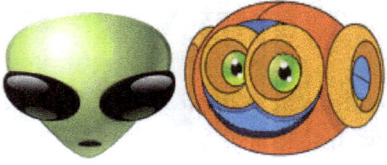

41. cosnuv	46. uncabeness
42. relhime	47. exyoded
43. defev	48. sanwixable
44. gaction	49. bufkibber
45. prefute	50. vomazful

The alien words test will show if the pupil can join together simple one-syllable words such as *cos* and *nuv* (from Alien Words Test 1) to make a multisyllabic word like *cosnuv*. Pupils who struggle with reading often won't be able to read multisyllabic words. They might be able to read *rain* and *coat*, but not *raincoat*. We need to show them how to do this. Struggler readers avoid multisyllabic words because they seem too long and hard to read, but in fact they are just composites of one-syllable words, or are made up of meaningful parts (morphemes); that is, prefix-, base word and -suffix, as in un-cabe-ness. We can teach students how to break such words into smaller parts in order to make the words easier to read (see Chapter 7 on teaching reading).

Problem: Unable to read multi-syllable words

For example, the student reads as follows:

Test word	Pupil's response
cosnuv	closttov
relhime	rever
sanwixable	sun…

Solutions:
- Try the syllable breaking lesson in Appendix 8
- Take words from a Big Book or enlarged text that you are reading to the class. For example, *The King's Birthday* has "maybe", "birthday" "opened", "pointing", "Friday". Divide the words into syllables and read the words out slowly phoneme by phoneme, as in: m-ay/b-e, b-ir-th/d-ay, o/p-e-n-ed, p-oi-n-t/i-ng, F-r-i/d-ay.

Assessment measures

READING

Step 1 Reading comprehension

Check whether the pupil is reading below their year level.

Informal measures

   1. Classroom "Running Records"

The running records procedure is described in Clay (2000, 2005). It involves the pupil reading classroom text with follow-up questions.

   2. PROBE reading test (Parkin & Parkin, 2011)

It is scored using the running records procedure. It consists of passages the student reads aloud and is scored like a running record, with follow-up reading comprehension questions. It also can be used as a listening comprehension measure.

Standardised measures

   1. *PAT: Reading* (Darr, McDowall, Ferral, Twist, & Watson, 2008) (NZCER)

This is a New Zealand-normed test that assesses reading comprehension and vocabulary from Years 3 to 10. The student reads passages silently and answers questions about them. It gives stanines (levels 1–9) to show reading levels (an average or better reader will be rated as stanine 5–9).

   2. *STAR Test* (NZCER, 2014)

This is a New Zealand-normed test. It assesses reading comprehension at the sentence and paragraph level. It also assesses decoding and vocabulary knowledge. Its coverage is Years 3–9. The student completes four sections: decoding (where they circle the word that matches a picture), sentence understanding (where they circle a word that fits into a sentence), paragraph comprehension (where they choose a word that fits the sense of the passage), and vocabulary (where they choose a word that fits a certain sentence meaning). The test reports stanines.

3. *Neale Analysis of Reading Ability (NARA)* (Neale, McKay, & Barnard, 1999).
This test assesses passage reading accuracy, reading comprehension and speed of reading from Year 1 to Year 7. It is normed in Australia and the UK. The student reads passages aloud, and they are scored for accuracy and speed. The student answers comprehension questions after each passage. The test provides percentiles, stanines and reading ages.

4. *York Assessment of Reading Comprehension (YARC)* (GL Assessment, 2012).
This test assesses passage reading accuracy, reading comprehension and reading rate. Its coverage is Year 1 to Year 9. It is normed in Australia and the UK. It has the same format as the NARA. It gives standard scores and reading ages.

5. *Wide Range Achievement Test (WRAT)* (Wilkinson, 2006)
This test assesses sentence comprehension. It also assesses word reading, spelling and maths. It is normed in the US. Coverage is from Year 1 to high school level. The test of word reading involves reading a list of graded words. The spelling test involves spelling words taken from a graded list. The sentence comprehension test uses sentences, where the student reads the sentences and answers questions about them. It gives percentiles, standard scores, stanines, and grade levels.

Step 2 Listening comprehension?

Check if the student is below average in listening comprehension.

Informal measures

An informal way to assess listening comprehension is to use graded reading materials suitable for the pupil's age level, but instead read them aloud to the pupil and ask comprehension questions, or ask them to recite the passage back to you. You then make a judgement as to whether they understand the material. PROBE passages (see the test description above) can be used in this way: you read a passage that is at the student's age level aloud to the pupil and ask the comprehension questions that go with the passage.

Standardised measures

1. *PAT Listening Comprehension* (NZCER, 2010)
This is a New Zealand-normed test. Its coverage is Year 3 to Year 10. The student listens to recorded passages and answers questions about them. It gives scale scores and stanines.

2. *Peabody Picture Vocabulary Test (PPVT)* (Dunn & Dunn, 2007a)
This test is standardised in the US. It is a test of receptive vocabulary. The student looks at a page with illustrations on it and chooses the illustration that fits the test item; for

example, "Point to the picture of angry". Its coverage is Year 1 to adult level. It gives percentiles, stanines and a language age.

   3. *British Picture Vocabulary Scale (BPVS)* (Dunn & Dunn, 2007b)
This test is standardised in the UK. It is the British version of PPVT. It also gives stanines and a language age.

Step 3 Word Reading Skills—Decoding

Check if the pupil is below average in decoding as measured by an oral reading test that can be a word reading test or a test of passage reading accuracy or a non-word test. A word or passage reading test is not a pure measure of decoding because there will be irregularly spelled words that are "sight" words and in passage reading the result is affected by use of context cues, but it does not seem to matter too much in that all these measures are good predictors as they correlate highly with a non-word reading test. A "pure" measure of decoding is a non-word test.

Standardised tests of word reading

   1. *Burt Word Reading Test* (Gilmore, Croft, & Reid, 1981): see Appendix 1A.
This is a normed New Zealand test of ability to read a list of words graded from easy to difficult. Its coverage is from Year 2 to Year 7. It gives reading ages.

   2. *STAR Test* (NZCER, 2014) has a subtest for word recognition. It gives stanines to show reading level.

   3. *Wide Range Achievement Test* (WRAT) (Wilkinson, 2006) assesses word recognition from Year 1 to high school level. It is a list of words graded from easy to difficult. It is normed in the US. It gives percentiles, stanines, and grade levels.

Tests of oral reading accuracy using texts or text passages

   1. Classroom "Running Records"
The running records procedure is described in Clay (2000, 2005). It involves the pupil reading classroom text aloud and gives an indication of decoding skill.

   2. *PROBE reading test* (Parkin & Parkin, 2011)
It is scored using the running records procedure. It asks pupils to read passage aloud like a running record. It gives an indication of decoding skill.

   3. *Neale Analysis of Reading Ability (NARA)* (Neale, McKay, & Barnard, 1999)
This 50-item test assesses passage reading accuracy from Year 1 to Year 6. It indicates decoding skill.

Non-word reading tests

A direct test of decoding skill, without context clues or memory to help the pupil, is to use non-words or "alien" words. These can only be pronounced by sounding out the words.

Standardised tests of non-word reading

   1. *Martin and Pratt Non-Word Reading Test* (Martin & Pratt, 2001)
This test is for ages 6–16 years. It is an Australian test. It gives reading ages.

   2. *Graded Non Word Reading Test* (Snowling, Sothard, & McLean, 1996).
This test is normed from Year 2 to Year 6 and gives reading ages. It is a UK test.

Informal tests of non-word reading

Bryant Test of Basic Decoding Skills (Bryant, 1975): see this chapter and Appendix 1B. It has a list of 20 three-letter words (e.g., maz), five words that assess the "silent e" rule (e.g., "fut<u>e</u>"), five words that assess consonant digraphs (e.g., <u>cho</u>), 10 words that assess consonant blends and vowel digraphs (e.g., "g<u>roaf</u>") and 10 words that assess multi-syllable decoding (e.g., "cos/nuv").

Writing

Step 1 Ideas

Informal measures

You can assess writing ideas using Ministry of Education writing exemplars: http://assessment.tki.org.nz/Assessment-tools-resources/The-New-Zealand-Curriculum-Exemplars

There are also National Standards exemplars: http://literacyonline.tki.org.nz/Literacy-Online/Student-needs/National-Standards-Reading-and-Writing/National-Standards-illustrations

For explanation of the exemplars see McLachlan, Nicholson, Fielding-Barnsley, Mercer, and Ohi (2013).

Standardised measures of writing—assessing ideas

   1. *Test of Written Language (TOWL 4)* (Hammill & Larsen, 2009)
This test is for students aged 9–17 years. It has a section that involves the student writing a story. There are picture stimuli on a topic (e.g., a storm, an accident). For writing mechanics, the story is scored on criteria such as number of sentences, paragraphing,

and so on. For quality of writing, the pupil's story is rated on whether it has an engaging beginning, has a story structure (characters, plot, setting) and an engaging ending. It is normed in the US. It gives percentiles.

> 2. *Test of Early Written Language (TEWL 3)* (Hresko, Herron, Peak, & Hicks, 2012)

This test is for pupils aged 4–11 years. This is a similar assessment to the one above but for younger pupils. It is normed in the US.

Step 2 Spelling

Informal assessment

An informal measure of spelling for beginner or struggle spellers is the invented spelling test. See Appendix 1E.

Standardised tests of spelling

> 1. *Wide Range Achievement Test (WRAT)* (Wilkinson, 2006)

This is a standardised test and assesses spelling of words. It is a graded list of words and is normed from kindergarten up to high school level. It gives percentiles, standard scores, and stanines. It can be given as an individual or group test.

> 2. *PRETOS (Proof Reading Tests of Spelling)* (Croft, Gilmore, Reid, & Jackson, 1981)

This test asks the pupil to choose the correct spelling from several options. It is for ages 8–13 years. It can be given as an individual or group test so can use it for the whole class. It has percentile scores.

> 3. *Progressive achievement tests in written spelling, punctuation, and grammar (PAT-SPG)* (ACER Press, 2011).

This test is normed for Years 2–10. It is an Australian test. It reports percentiles and stanines. It can be given as an individual or group test.

Note: If these reading and spelling tests are unavailable to you, you may wish to do an Internet search for the Schonell Reading and Spelling tests (Schonell, 1950). They are easy to use and you can download the tests. They are normed for Years 1–6.

Further testing: assessing problems with pre-reading skills

A student with dyslexia may need further assessment of their pre-reading skills, especially if they are in the early years of school. The pre-reading skills of knowing the alphabet names and sounds and having phoneme awareness—even at a simple level, such as being able to break words into syllables or knowing the first sound in "fish", or being able to tell you a word that rhymes with fish—are both highly predictive of later reading development. Students who lack pre-reading skills at school entry often struggle with reading and writing.

Alphabet knowledge test—see Appendix 1C

Check that the pupil knows the names and sounds of the letters of the alphabet (Clay, 1993; Nicholson, 2005b). To crack the code they need to know the phonemes that correspond to each letter of the alphabet. Some letters represent two phonemes; for example, the sound of *x* has two phonemes /ks/ and so does *q*—it has two phonemes /kw/. They may have trouble with reversible letters like *b* and *d*. These can be easily taught: a good technique is to teach how to make the shape of a bed by clenching the fingers of each hand but leaving the thumb facing up and then putting each hand together to make the shape of a bed. If they look at the shape starting from the left, and think of its first sound, /b/, then they will see the thumb and the clenched fingers of the left hand making the shape of the *b* and know how to read/spell it. The other end of the bed has the clenched fingers and thumb making the shape of the *d*.

Phonemic Awareness Test—see Appendix 2

This phonemic awareness test (Nicholson, 2005a, 2005b; Roper, 1984) assesses the pupil's ability to blend phonemes together to make a word, count phonemes in words, take off phonemes, and add phonemes to spoken words. Use the chart (make sure the pupil does not see it) to ask each question and keep a score of correct and incorrect responses, writing down the incorrect ones so that you can get an idea of what they are thinking when they answer. A copy of the GKR phonemic awareness test is in Appendix 1D.

The test is a check for phonemic awareness; that is, awareness of the smallest distinct sounds in words. To crack the code, pupils need to know how to break spoken words into phonemes. When they are able to do this, they can relate letters of the alphabet to their sounds and connect these to printed words.

English has 40 or so phonemes: not just the 21 consonants and five long vowel sounds, but others as well, such as *ch*, *sh* and *th*, and diphthongs such as *ew* as in *few* and *ow* as in *cow*. The pupil needs to be aware of these sounds in spoken words. A phonemic awareness assessment does not involve reading. What you do is say the word and the pupil answers questions you ask about how to break the word into sounds.

Diagnostic information

An important indicator of beginning skill in phonemic awareness is blending (the ability to recognise a spoken word if you say it slowly) and segmentation (the ability to tell you what phonemes are in a word—see the test in Appendix 1D). If the pupil can blend phonemes in spoken words and work out the word then they can do this for reading as well when they decode it phoneme by phoneme. Segmentation is the ability to tell you the separate phonemes in the word and this skill is important also for reading and spelling. If the pupil can mentally break the word into its phonemes then they are aware that words are made of small units of sound and this is the insight they need for reading and spelling. If they can break off the initial or final sound of a spoken word this is good to know. It means they will be able to work out the initial and end sounds of words. Substitution skills are sophisticated; they indicate the pupil can manipulate sounds in words and they could do this in reading and spelling as well, noticing alliteration and rimes when they compare similarly spelled words.

Summary

When you assess a pupil for dyslexia, be sure to focus on the positive. Assessment is not about deficit thinking. It is about assessing strengths. Remember that the student with dyslexia may have problems with spelling and pronouncing words when reading them, but they can be very engaging in terms of language and ideas. Look for these strengths while you are assessing.

This chapter has explained the steps you can take to decide if the student has dyslexia. We did this by explaining that the student with dyslexia is likely to have good oral language skills but to be weak in their ability to crack the code. The chapter has provided some ideas for gathering diagnostic data to find out what exactly is confusing the dyslexic student when decoding unfamiliar words.

PART FOUR
TACKLING DYSLEXIA

CHAPTER 7

Teaching children with dyslexia to read

Introduction

There is little debate that good reading and writing skills are essential for academic success. We also know that not all children achieve good reading and writing skills, and that for some children this is due to being dyslexic. The simple view of reading (Gough & Tunmer, 1986) categorises dyslexia as one of three types of reading difficulties. This group of readers have good language comprehension but poor decoding skills. Decoding difficulties are preventing these readers from becoming good readers. Children with reading difficulties can also have difficulty with language comprehension, or both decoding and language comprehension.

Although the most common type of reading difficulty is poor decoding *and* poor language comprehension, we also know that up to 10 percent of the population are poor decoders with good language comprehension (i.e., dyslexic). In Chapter 1 we discussed the nature of dyslexia and the fact that there are degrees of dyslexia. Some students with dyslexia may display a mild form, while others are severe. It is possible that some New Zealand classrooms may not have students with dyslexia while the classroom next door may have a number of students with dyslexia.

Hopefully by now you will be able to identify students with dyslexia, or at least screen for dyslexia (refer to Chapter 6). But another challenge for classroom teachers is to know how to develop the reading skills of students with dyslexia. This chapter begins by discussing research on the characteristics of effective reading tutoring programmes. We also outline the decoding strategies and understanding of the English language that good readers need to acquire. We briefly discuss comprehension and vocabulary strategies, but our greatest emphasis is on decoding, because this is the main stumbling block for students with dyslexia when learning to read. Three mini case studies are then presented.

The characteristics of effective tutoring programmes

Tutoring can be part of the everyday classroom, as in peer tutoring, where better readers in the classroom assist poor readers, or cross-age tutoring, where older students in the school tutor younger students; or where the teacher takes time in class or out of class to tutor a small group or an individual student. Juel's (1996) review of tutoring programmes in the US identified four characteristics of effective interventions:
- tutor modelling and explaining
- scaffolded instruction in word reading and spelling (i.e. with the tutor teaching reading and spelling so that it is not too hard or easy and gives support)
- explicit instruction in letter–sound relationships
- instruction at the word level (i.e. teaching how to read words in isolation and in context).

Bennett's (2009) New Zealand study of effective tutors of reading focused on the strategies tutors use to develop good readers, the observed characteristics of effective tutors, and the characteristics the effective tutors themselves believed they had. The effective tutors in Bennett's study spent a significant proportion of the weekly hour-long sessions teaching letter–sound relationships, raising phonemic awareness and listening to the children read. These tutors also used both open and closed questions, praise and scaffolded instruction; maintained high levels of engaged learning; reversed roles (i.e. the child taught the tutor strategies they had been learning); and helped their students through telling, demonstrating, directing and questioning. The tutors kept students motivated by using reward charts and reading logs, providing short breaks, maintaining routines, using hands-on materials (such as magnetic letters, flip cards, individual whiteboards), selecting reading material that was relevant to the interests of the child, and at times allowing the children to select their own reading book/reader to read aloud from.

Bennett (2009) reported that the effective tutors in her study were also:
- good communicators
- able to build positive relationships
- flexible
- consistent with routines
- reflective
- knowledgeable and experienced.

The tutors in Bennett's (2009) study were asked to identify what they believed to be the characteristics of effective reading tutors. She found a close relationship between observed characteristics and perceived characteristics. The perceived characteristics included:
- a positive tutor–child relationship
- being flexible
- the ability to gain and maintain the child's attention
- a good understanding of the child's reading skills
- a good knowledge of the reading process and the skills to teach reading strategies
- gathering assessment data to inform teaching
- the ability to communicate with the child.

Matthew effects in reading interventions

Research suggests that there are Matthew effects (Stanovich, 1986; 2000) in remedial reading interventions. The term 'Matthew effects', after the Gospel of Matthew, is used to describe the impact of reading on vocabulary and comprehension. The concept of Matthew effects is where readers who get off to a good start in reading read more which further enhances their vocabulary and reading comprehension: that is, the rich get richer. Readers who do not get off to a good start in reading read less, if at all, reducing their opportunities to build vocabulary and reading comprehension: that is, the poor get poorer. Data from 190 struggling readers showed that students who were significantly behind in reading did not gain as much from one-to-one interventions as students who were not as far behind in reading (Nicholson & Dymock, 2011). The 190 students, aged from 5 to 15 years, all reading below age level (based on a battery of standardised reading measures), were placed into two groups: 'skilled' poor readers and 'less skilled' poor readers. Placement in one of the two groups was based on pre-test reading stanine scores.[1] Students with stanine scores of 4 or above were placed in the skilled poor reader group; students with stanine scores below 4 were placed in the less skilled poor reader group.

The *Neale Analysis of Reading Ability* (Neale et al., 1999), a standardised measure, was used to measure reading accuracy and reading comprehension, both prior to the intervention and afterwards. Other measures were used to assess reading-related skills and knowledge, such as phonemic awareness (Nicholson, 2005a) and receptive vocabulary (Dunn & Dunn, 2007a). The year-long intervention focused on developing phonological awareness, decoding strategies, reading high-frequency words, reading connected text, comprehension, and spelling strategies. Following the reading intervention, assessment results showed that the skilled poor reader group made greater gains in both reading accuracy and reading comprehension than the less skilled poor reader group. Put another way, the rich (or skilled poor readers) got richer and the poorer (or less skilled poor readers) remained poor. The gains between the two groups of readers in both accuracy and comprehension were significantly different.

Figure 7.1 shows the rate of progress in reading accuracy, over an academic year, for the 190 children. This illustrates clearly that the rich did get richer, and that the poor remained poor.

---

1 Stanine is a scale that breaks the curve into nine categories, or stanines. Stanine 1 is well below average, stanine 9 is excellent, and stanine 5 is average.

Figure 7.1: Reading accuracy rate of progress (in stanines)

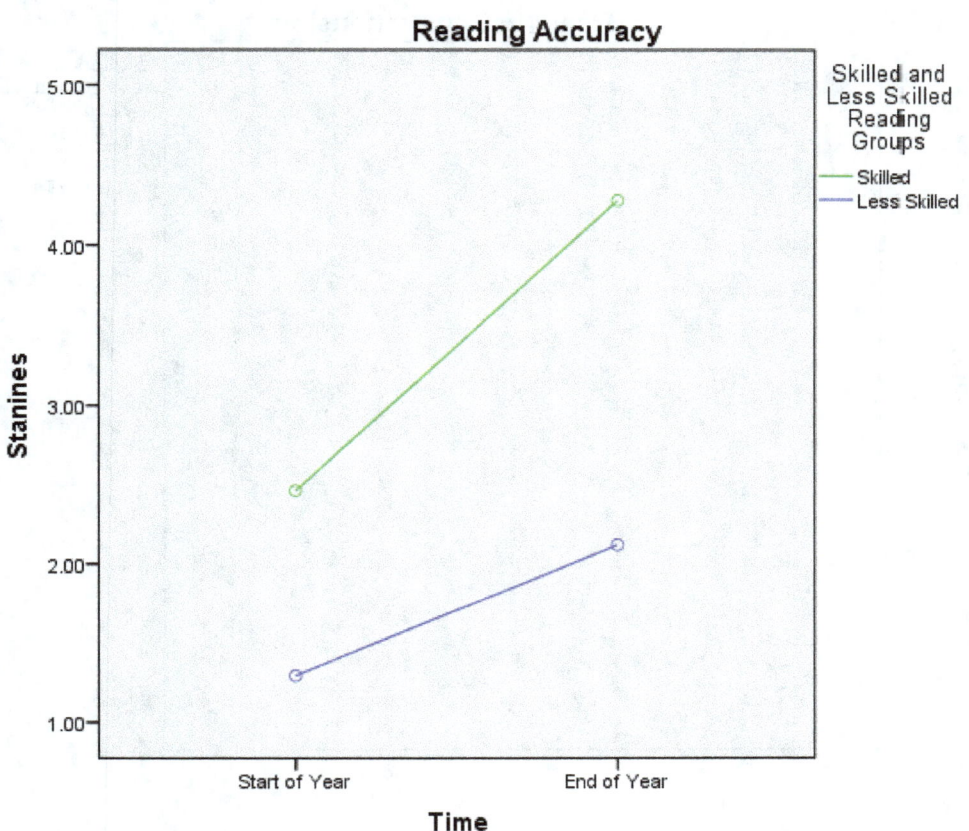

Source: Nicholson and Dymock (2011). Graph has been adapted slightly.

Figure 7.2 shows the rate of progress in reading *comprehension* for the 190 students over the academic year. Again, the results show Matthew effects (Stanovich, 1986; 2000), whereby the rich get richer and the poor remain poor.

Figure 7.2: Reading comprehension rate of progress (in stanines)

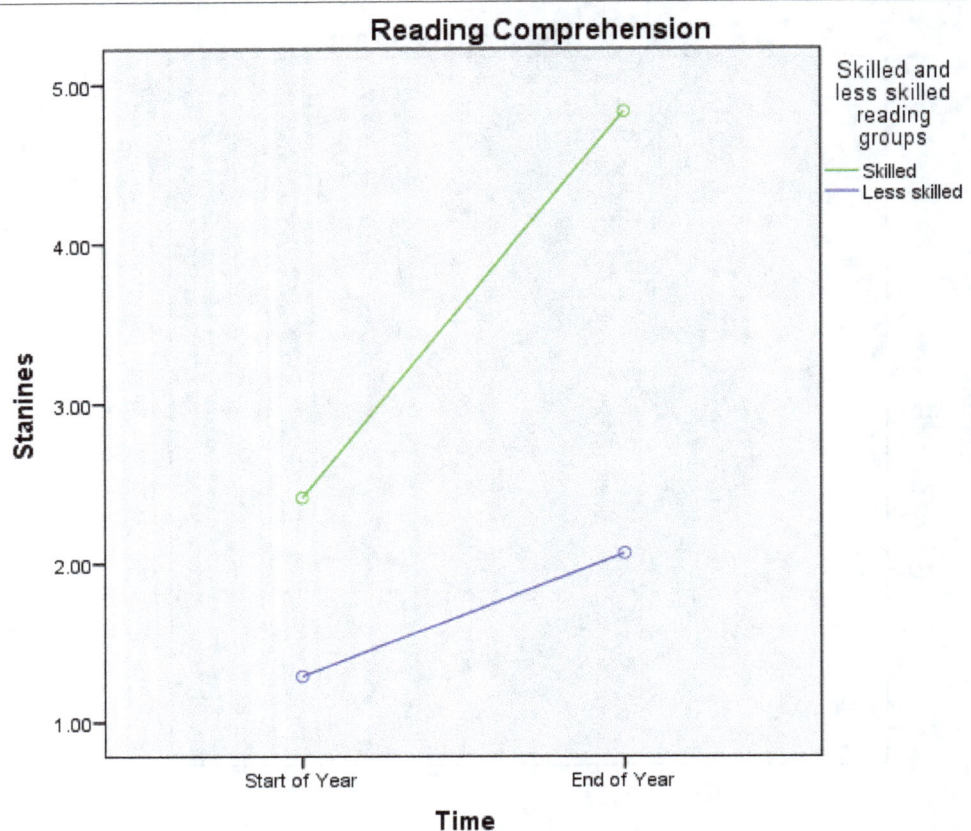

Source: Nicholson and Dymock (2011). Graph has been adapted slightly.

The findings suggest that there are Matthew effects in reading interventions (Stanovich, 1986; 2000). The differences in both reading accuracy and reading comprehension of poor readers when commencing an intervention will benefit pupils who begin the intervention with higher levels of reading skills (that is, the poor readers who are close to average). Poor but more-skilled readers will gain more from the intervention, in terms of gains in accuracy and comprehension, than poor less-skilled readers. Nicholson and Dymock (2011) propose that the key factor is not the intervention itself (as less-skilled poor readers did make gains), but rather the intensity of the programme. Less-skilled poor readers may require a higher frequency or "higher dosage of instruction" (Nicholson & Dymock, 2011, p. 32; refer also to Torgesen, 2000; Al Otaiba & Fuchs, 2006). For certain groups of readers, Nicholson and Dymock (2011) recommend more intensive instruction at the beginning of instruction. The results also suggest the importance of early assessment and intervention—*before* the gap between chronological and reading age becomes large.

This element of time and intensity means that, in the classroom, less-skilled readers will need more time and direct instruction covering less material than the proficient group—perhaps half as much material and twice as much time, with adjustments—so that the teaching is not too hard or too easy. Implementing it in the classroom takes knowledge and organisational skill, as well as administrative support. If tutoring or other assistance is occurring, it makes sense that classroom instruction to some degree co-ordinates with the extra help, otherwise the student who needs more time on less material ends up getting more material to cover with no more time.

There are a number of implications for teachers and tutors that stem from studies such as those done by Juel (1996), Bennett (2009) and Nicholson and Dymock (2011). The findings provide a useful checklist for teachers and tutors. For example, 'Am I flexible?', 'Am I consistent with routines?', 'Do I have a good understanding of the reading process and the strategies readers need to learn?', 'Am I able to interpret assessment data and develop a plan that meets the student's needs?' and 'Is the intervention intensive enough for the reader?'

One implication of the research is that effective tutors must have the necessary knowledge to assess, plan and implement a suitable intervention that meets the needs of the student with dyslexia. Knowledge about language and reading strategies, particularly decoding, is a major challenge for children with dyslexia. In the following section we will discuss the characteristics of good readers, which will assist in determining what knowledge and skills readers with dyslexia need to gain.

Decoding strategies, including knowledge of the English language, needed to become a good reader

What skills do good readers have? According to the simple view of reading, reading is the product of decoding and language comprehension. That is, good readers are good decoders and have good language comprehension. A good reader also has a large vocabulary. A strength of the simple view is that, as we have seen, it also identifies three types of reading disability:

- difficulty with *decoding* (but good language comprehension)
- difficulty with *language comprehension* (but good decoding)
- difficulty with both *decoding and language comprehension*.

Treatment resisters

Poor decoding skills, in terms of both accuracy and fluency, are the primary stumbling block for children with dyslexia. Typically these children are 'treatment resisters' (Torgesen, 2000). Treatment resisters do not consciously resist treatment; rather, they don't make sufficient progress and gains relative to the effort they put in. In other words, treatment resisters are fully engaged in the intervention, receptive and keen to learn, yet progress is very slow.

The research is quite clear on the *type* of intervention children with dyslexia need (refer to Bennett, 2009; Juel, 1996; Nicholson & Dymock, 2011; Shaywitz, 2003). However, we have yet to reach a consensus on "how much of that instruction, delivered under what conditions, will lead to adequate development of word reading and passage comprehension skills in children with phonological processing weaknesses" (Torgesen, 2000, p. 63). By phonological processing weaknesses we mean difficulty in breaking spoken sentences into words, words into syllables and syllables into phonemes. An important message is, don't give up. It is better to be positive and take the stand that "all children *can* be taught to read" (Shaywitz, 2003, p. 169).

Even though this is the ideal we all want for the student with dyslexia—that they will be taught to read—the practicalities of school instruction and limited resources often mean that both teacher and student run out of time. At some point content trumps decoding and reading instruction, and therefore teachers must, as needed, provide other non-reading access for students who can't 'read it' in order to avoid double jeopardy (being punished twice for the same offence). This means giving access to alternative ways of getting the content without having to read the material. Examples might be talking books, YouTube, speech-to-text functions on the computer, other videos of the subject matter, illustrations to show the nature of the content to be learned, and so on. This is especially important for the dyslexic student.

Decoding strategies

Phonological awareness

In order to develop decoding strategies, the reader must have a degree of *phonological awareness*: they must know letter names and the sounds they represent, and have an understanding of the layers of English. 'Phonological awareness' is an umbrella term for awareness of levels of speech sound, including syllables, onset-rimes and phonemes (see Figure 7.3). Phonological awareness has nothing to do with print. It is an awareness of the sounds in language at the syllable, onset-rime and phoneme level (see Figure 7.3 and the following explanatory text).

Figure 7.3: Phonological awareness

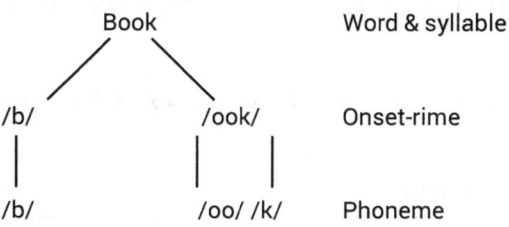

> *Syllable:* "A unit of sequential speech sounds containing a vowel and any consonants preceding or following that vowel" (Henry, 2010, p. 314).
> *Onset-rime:* The onset is the initial consonant or consonants within a syllable. The rime is the vowel and any consonant that follows, within the syllable.
> *Phoneme*: "The smallest unit of sound that conveys a distinction in meaning" (Henry, 2010, p. 312). A phoneme is the smallest sound unit that can change the meaning of a word. In the English language there are between 40 to 46 phonemes, and these phonemes are represented by 26 letters.[2] In English the 40 to 46 phonemes produce over 500,000 words.

[2] The general consensus is that there are 40 English phonemes but due to dialect differences estimates vary and can be up to 46.

Phonemic awareness

Phonemic awareness is "The insight that spoken words are made up of a sequence of somewhat separable sounds" (Graves, Juel, & Graves, 2004, p. 93) and "the ability to manipulate sounds in words" (Henry, 2010, p. 312). Phonemic awareness is an awareness of the minimal unit of sound in language. It is an insight into speech. Phonemic awareness is not phonics, or knowing which sound goes with which letter.

Phonemic awareness is a critical first step in learning the alphabetic principle: letters on their own or in words represent little speech sounds we call phonemes (e.g., s=/s/ as in *sun*, f=/f/ as in *frog*, a=/a/ as in *app*).

Phonemic awareness is important for learning to read because it helps children to understand the alphabetic principle and that English is an alphabetic language (i.e., letters represent sounds in writing). In English, phonemes are represented by letters and letter clusters. In order to understand the way that oral language is represented by print (i.e., letters), children must understand that the words in their oral language are composed of small segments of sound. That is, for a child to learn that the letter *m* makes a /m/ sound, as in "mouse" the child must have a level of phonemic awareness. If there is a limited or no level of awareness, the child does not understand that the letter *m* makes an /m/ sound. Children who lack phonemic awareness have serious difficulty learning to read and write (Adams, 1990; Nicholson, 2005a).

Layers of English

There are three distinct layers of English: Anglo-Saxon, Latin and Greek, as shown in Figure 7.4.

Figure 7.4: The layers of English

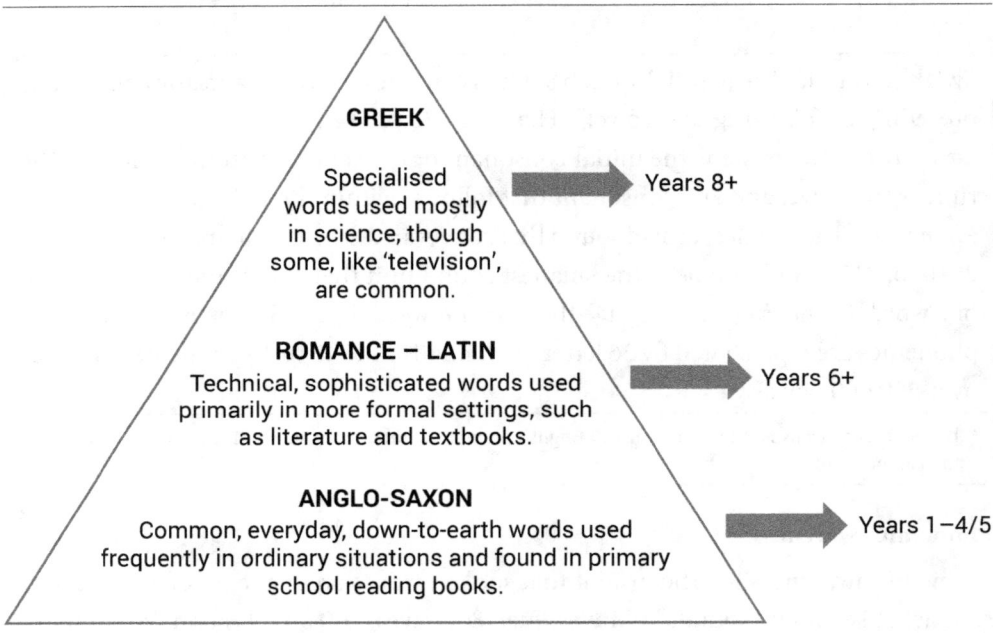

Source: Calfee & Associates, 1984

The **Anglo-Saxon layer**, the largest layer of English, consists of common, everyday words that all speakers of English use (e.g., *the, is, it, at, day, hat, mother, father*). Anglo-Saxon words usually have only one or two syllables. Approximately 43 percent of Anglo-Saxon syllables are 'closed' and follow a consonant-short-vowel-consonant (CVC) pattern. Words like *bat, fat, sit, cot, pet* and *put* are closed syllables, where the single vowel is followed by a consonant. Open syllables comprise 32 percent of Anglo-Saxon syllable patterns. In open syllables the vowel is at the end of the syllable, and the vowel is usually long (e.g., *bee, be, go, hi, she*). The remaining 25 percent of syllables are of 4 types: vowel-consonant-*e* (VCE) (e.g., *hate*); vowel digraph (e.g., *br**ea**d*); consonant-*le* (e.g., *tum**ble***); and *r*-controlled (e.g., *t**ur**n*) (Henry, 2010; Moats, 2000). Table 7.1 presents common Anglo-Saxon syllable patterns.

Table 7.1: Common Anglo-Saxon syllable patterns (and examples)

Syllable	Defined	Examples
Closed (CVC)	Single vowel is followed by a consonant	bat shut is rabbit (rab-bit)
Open (CV)	Vowel is at the end of the syllable. Vowel is usually long	bee hi go re-
Vowel-consonant-*e* (VCE)	Vowel is long (*e* is silent as it acts as a marker) This is called a "split digraph" in the UK	made time place cute
Vowel digraph	Sometimes referred to as a vowel team or vowel pair	rain boil
Consonant-*le*	Typically starts with a consonant that is part of the syllable (-gle, -ble)	stum-*ble*
r-controlled	Vowels are usually co-articulated with the *r*	bark mart

Notes:
Open and closed syllables = 75 percent of Anglo-Saxon syllables.
C = consonant; V = vowel

Closed syllables form a number of patterns, and these are shown in Table 7.2 (Goswami, n.d.). Table 7.2 also includes the syllable frequency of approximately 4,000 monosyllabic words (Goswami, n.d.).

Table 7.2: Closed syllable patterns

Closed syllable pattern	Examples	Percentage
CVC	cat hit	43
CVCC	desk best past	21
CCVC	trip	15
CCVCC	grasp	6

Source: Goswami, n.d.
Notes:
CV (open syllable) = 5 percent.
C = consonant; V = vowel.

There are more than 80 Anglo-Saxon decoding strategies. Decoding strategies, like comprehension strategies, are plans or tactics the reader uses to decode or comprehend text. Knowing that the letter 's' makes an /s/ sound rather than a /f/ or /t/ sound is a strategy the reader uses when they encounter the letter 's'. These strategies are summarised in Table 7.3. If students are making age-appropriate progress, they should have a good understanding of the Anglo-Saxon consonants and vowels by the end of Year 4, or by the age of 9.

Table 7.3: Anglo-Saxon consonants and vowels

Consonants		
Single	**Blends**	**Digraphs**
p g d b c v w l r t f j m n s h k q x y z	_Initial_ bl br cl cr dr fl fr gl gr sl pr tr sc sk scr spl sm squ sn str sp st sw tw thr _Final_ - ft -mp -nt -lk	_Initial_ ch sh th wh gh _Final_ -ng -ck -ch
Vowels		
Single Short Long	**r & l controlled**	**Digraphs**
a: mad made **e:** pet Pete **i:** Tim time **o:** hop hope hops hopes hopped hoped hopping hoping **u:** cut cute	**ar:** park lard harm **or:** for horn short **er:** her stern fern **ir:** bird thirst sir **ur:** fur church burn **al:** hall fall call halter falter walk talk	**one sound**: ai/ay pain, play ee meet ie piece oi/oy foil, toy oa boat au/aw laud, law ew few **two sounds**: ea breath, breathe ei seize eight oo cook noon ou round* soul ow cow snow

Source: Calfee & Patrick, 1995, p. 108.

Note: R-controlled (or *r*-influenced) vowel patterns: when a vowel is followed by an r, the r affects the sound of the vowel (compare bird/bid; hard/had).

* The /ow/ sound of ou as in round is by far the most common sound of ou when it's on its own. The exception is -ous but that is only when ou is followed by s. The /oe/ sound for ou as in soul is far less common as is the ou pattern in words such as 'you' and 'soup'. (Stanback, 1992).

Students begin encountering words from the Romance or **Latin** layer of English from about Year 5. The Latin or Romance layer consists of longer, multisyllabic words that are largely associated with content area reading. A signpost for Latin-based words is the prefix, Latin root and suffix. The Latin root carries the major meaning of the word, but prefixes also carry meaning. Words such as *destruction* or *disruption* are Latin-based words. Latin words may have a prefix and Latin root (disrupt) or Latin root and suffix (rupture) or prefix, Latin root and suffix (disruption).

Table 7.4: Examples of Latin prefixes, roots and suffixes

Prefix	Latin root	Suffix	Word
de-	-struc	-tion	destruction
dis-	-rupt	-tion	disruption

The Latin layer is characterised by three syllable patterns: closed (e.g., *rupt*), vowel-consonant-e (VCE) (e.g., *scribe*) and r-controlled (e.g., *port*). In the Latin layer, vowel digraphs are uncommon, and when they do appear they are often in suffixes (*-tion*, *-ian*).

The **Greek** layer of English is typically associated with the language of scholars and scientists. The terminology of modern science is formed from Greek, particularly in aeronautics, biochemistry, chemotherapy, and genetics (Henry, 2010). The Greek layer consists of two roots or two Greek combining forms, both carrying equal meaning (e.g., *psych+ology = psychology*; *hydro+phobia = hydrophobia*). There are two syllable types that are associated with the Greek layer: closed (e.g., *graph*) and open (e.g., *pho-to*). Greek letter–sound correspondences are similar to those in Anglo-Saxon but incorporate new ones:

- *ch* is pronounced /k/ (e.g., *chemistry, chromosome*)
- *ph* is pronounced /f/ (e.g., *photograph, chlorophyll*)
- *y* is pronounced /i/ (e.g., *chlorophyll*).

For most children, learning the decoding strategies of the different layers of English is a slow process. Henry's (2010, p. 9) continuum for decoding and spelling (see Figure 7.5) illustrates the development of decoding skill. The continuum begins with phonological awareness, then alphabet names and sounds, followed by the Anglo-Saxon layer of English. According to Henry (2010), it is not until the end of the first 3 or 4 years at school that readers and spellers have a good grasp of the Anglo-Saxon layer of English.

Figure 7.5: The decoding–spelling continuum

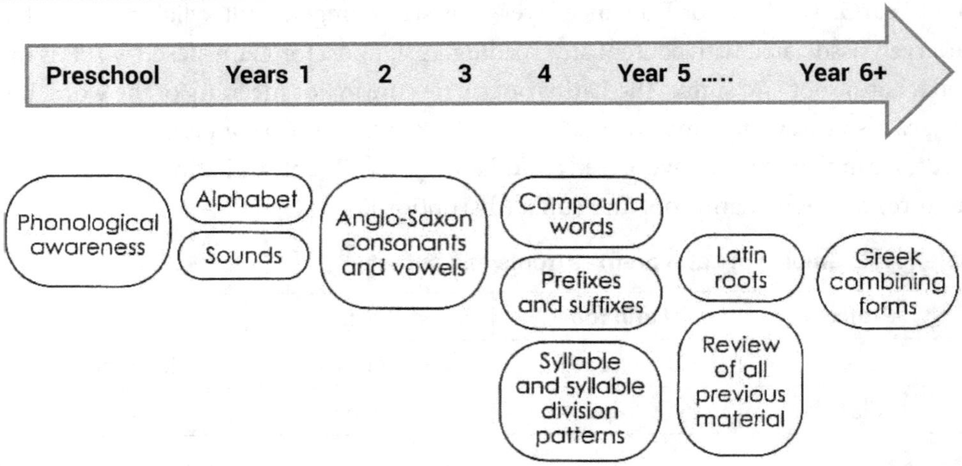

Preschool — Years 1 — 2 — 3 — 4 — Year 5 ..... — Year 6+

- Phonological awareness
- Alphabet
- Sounds
- Anglo-Saxon consonants and vowels
- Compound words
- Prefixes and suffixes
- Syllable and syllable division patterns
- Latin roots
- Review of all previous material
- Greek combining forms

Source: Henry, 2010, p. 9.

There is little debate that the English language is complex. Readers who have an understanding of the history of English will be at an advantage. The following YouTube clip by Kate Gardoqui provides an engaging explanation of how English evolved. The clip may be helpful when teaching your students about the English language.

http://www.youtube.com/watch?v=kIzFz9T5rhI

Also note the following two TED talks for spelling and decoding:

http://ed.ted.com/lessons/making-sense-of-spelling-gina-cooke

http://www.wordworkskingston.com/WordWorks/Orthographic_TED_Ed_Talks.html

Comprehension strategies

In this section we will provide a brief overview of comprehension strategy instruction. For a fuller account of teaching comprehension and accompanying lesson plans on how to teach comprehension strategies, refer to *Teaching Reading Comprehension: The What, the How, the Why* (Dymock & Nicholson, 2012).

Skilled readers use a number of comprehension strategies (Dymock & Nicholson, 2012). An important question teachers ask is, 'Which strategies should I teach?' The late Michael Pressley (2008), one of the field's most respected writers about comprehension, along with the National Institute of Child Health and Human Development (2000a) have recommended that teachers focus on just a small number of comprehension strategies that have strong research support. Pressley (2008, p. 606) calls for "complete teaching of a small repertoire of strategies, teaching through modelling and explanation, and scaffolded practice". We agree.

We recommend that teachers begin by teaching five key research-based comprehension strategies (Dymock & Nicholson, 2010; 2012). The five key strategies are:
(1) activating background knowledge;
(2) questioning;
(3) analysing text structure (e.g., narrative [story grammar] or expository text structures [text structure analysis or graphic organisers]);
(4) creating mental images; and
(5) summarising.

When students have a good understanding of the five strategies, teachers can add more to their repertoire. Due to the limited capacity of short-term memory, Miller (1956) warned against cognitive overload, or focusing on too much at any given time. We argue that it is better to keep it simple, taking advantage of the fact that the human mind can only hold up to seven (plus or minus two) pieces of information at one time (Miller, 1956). The High 5! bookmark shown in Figure 7.6 provides a useful reminder for students when they are reading. The strategies are described in more detail in the following text.

Figure 7.6: High 5! comprehension strategies

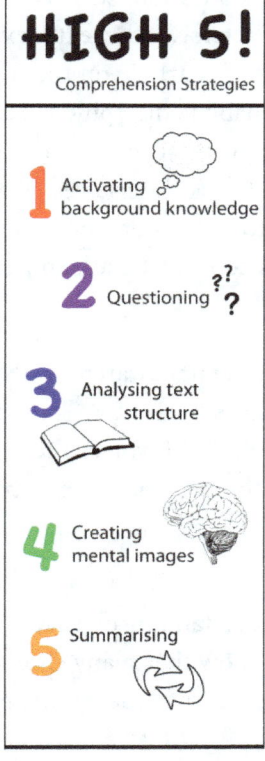

Activating background knowledge

Reading comprehension depends upon knowledge, and readers must activate this knowledge before comprehension can occur. Knowledge also builds knowledge. Activating prior knowledge or making connections to background knowledge involves the teacher asking open-ended questions that link directly to the content of the text, whereby students talk as much as, or more than, the teacher about their own experiences (Brown, 2002; Pressley, 2002). Initial questioning by the teacher can quickly establish if students lack the essential knowledge base. Background knowledge can then be built prior to reading (Stanovich, 2000). Students should also be taught to activate their background knowledge before, and during, reading, activating background knowledge on text structure and the content.

Questioning

Readers should be encouraged to generate and answer questions before and during reading, because this aids comprehension (Block & Parris, 2008; Block & Pressley, 2007; Dymock & Nicholson, 2012; National Reading Panel, 2000a). Prior to reading, good readers ask themselves questions that activate background knowledge. For example, good readers consider the text structure the writer has followed. If the text is narrative in structure, good readers will ask questions such as, 'Where and when does the story take place?' and 'Who are the characters?'. If the text is expository in structure, good readers will ask questions such as, 'Is this article on the monarch butterfly a descriptive text (e.g., describes the butterfly's habitat, diet, physical characteristics, unique features) or a sequential text (e.g., explains the life-cycle)?' If the article is sequential, readers should be encouraged, as they read, to ask themselves what will happen next. If the article is descriptive, focusing on one topic, readers should ask themselves as they read what the sub-topics are. Good readers continually ask and answer questions as they read.

Analysing text structure

Text structure awareness is a mental awareness of how writers organise information. Meyer and Rice (1984, p. 319) explain it as "how the ideas in a text are interrelated to convey a message to a reader." It involves the reader looking mentally for the text structure. Students encounter two main text structures in school: narrative and expository (non-fiction).

Narrative text

Most children have a basic understanding of narratives (i.e. beginning, middle and end), but research and experience show that many children are unaware that stories have a more elaborate structure (i.e. setting, characters, plot and theme) (Calfee & Patrick,

1995; Dymock & Nicholson, 2012). It is this more elaborate structure that children should be taught so that they can analyse narratives to enhance their comprehension. As Calfee and Patrick (1995) state,

> Instruction in the narrative domain leads students to a deeper understanding of how narratives are built, and gives them technical language for talking about both comprehension and composition. (p. 77)

When reading narratives, students should be taught:
- that the *setting* establishes where and when the story takes place
- that *characters* can be classified as major and minor
- how to analyse individual *characters*, focusing on their appearance and personality, and how to compare and contrast characters
- how to analyse the overall *plot*—the plot consists of four parts:
  - problem (What is the problem in the story?)
  - response (How do character/s respond to the problem?)
  - action (What do characters do about the problem?)
  - outcome (What is the outcome?)
- how to analyse individual episodes (i.e. sub-plots)—diagrams can be used to enable the reader to visualise the episode analysis
- that the *theme* is the message that underlies the story—the theme often explains the motives of the characters, or comments on social relationships, or society in general; the theme is often left to the reader to interpret, so ask your pupils, 'Why did the author write the story?'

A story web can be also be created. A story web is like a word web where the terms defining the structure of a story surround the title (see Figure 7.7).

Figure 7.7: A story web structure

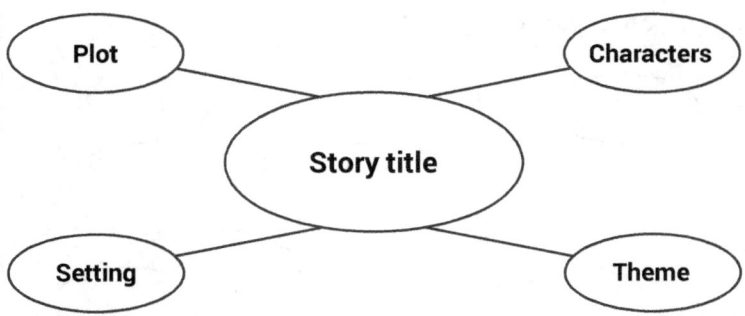

Expository text

Expository or non-fiction text has many types of structure, and some are very complex. Exposition can be separated into two broad groups: texts that describe and texts that are affected by time (Calfee & Patrick, 1995). Within these two broad groups we have found that students typically encounter six expository text types—three descriptive and three sequential.

Descriptive texts

These texts present the attributes of something (e.g., the attributes of New York City, the kakapo, or citrus fruit). The three most common descriptive text patterns are *list*, *web* and *matrix*. The most basic descriptive pattern is the list. This may be a shopping list, a list of countries that grow sugar cane, or, in science, the polar bears' diet (e.g., seals, carcasses of whales and walruses). With a list it doesn't matter what goes first. Figure 7.8 shows a list pattern.

Figure 7.8: A list pattern for descriptive text

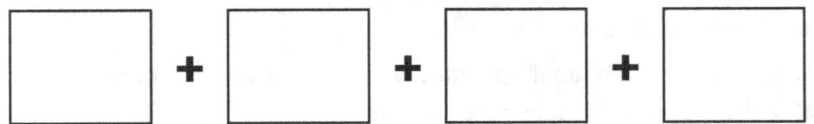

The *web* is the simplest writing structure for informational articles. This text structure is named a web because it resembles a spider's web (Calfee & Patrick, 1995). A spider-web has a centre and a number of fine threads that form a network of lines. In the web, the attributes of an object are discussed and the attributes have a common link. For example, the article may be discussing the characteristics of the red deer (e.g., diet, habitat, physical characteristics, enemies) or the features of San Francisco (e.g., tourism, economy, education, history). Figure 7.9 shows a web pattern.

Figure 7.9: A web pattern for descriptive text

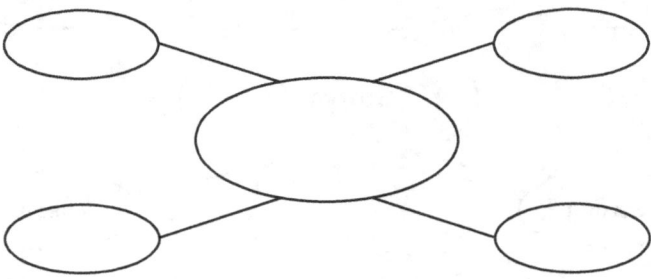

Finally, a *matrix* compares and contrasts two or more topics. For example, the author may be comparing brown, black and polar bears, types of roses, bicycles (e.g., mountain, road and BMX), or hatchback cars. Figure 7.10 shows a matrix pattern.

Figure 7.10: A matrix pattern for descriptive text

Sequential texts

These texts present a series of events which progresses over time. Normally, sequential texts are set out in a first-to-last pattern. The three more common sequential structures are the string, cause–effect, and problem–solution. The string is where a chronological description of events is given (e.g., the sequence involved in making pikelets, or the step-by-step process from the time peonies are picked in a New Zealand field to the moment they arrive in a New York City flower shop). Or it could refer to a sequence to follow in working out a maths problem, or the sequence beavers follow in building a dam. Figure 7.11 shows a string pattern.

Figure 7.11: A string pattern for sequential text

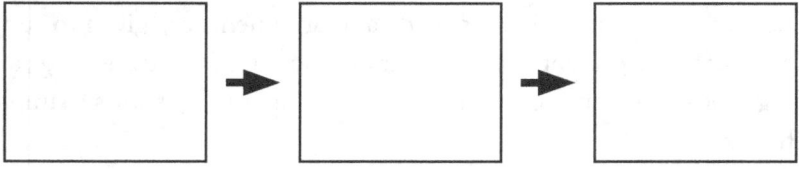

In cause–effect texts, two or more ideas or events interact with one another. One is the cause and the other the effect or results. Cause-effect is different to a string in that cause-effect implies one thing causes another whereas in a string it is not necessarily like that. For example the steps in baking a cake is a string of actions one after the other but they are not actions that cause something to happen as would be the case in a cause-effect pattern such as losing control of your bicycle causing you to fall off, or the causes and effects of acid rain, or the 2011 *Rena* oil spill. This pattern is common in history, science and health publications. A cause–effect pattern is shown below. Figure 7.12 shows a cause-effect pattern.

Figure 7.12: A cause–effect pattern for sequential text

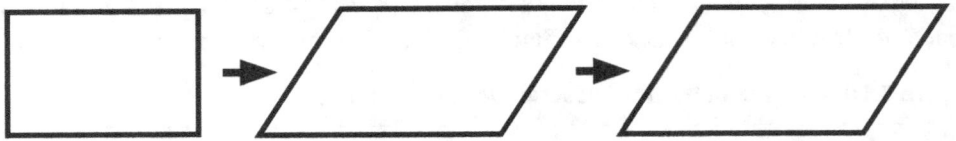

In problem–solution texts, the authors state a problem or pose a question, followed by a solution or answer in the text (e.g., a problem associated with leaky homes, or poverty, or school bullying). Figure 7.13 shows a problem–solution pattern.

Figure 7.13: A problem–solution pattern for descriptive text

Problems	Solutions
1.	1.
2.	2.
3.	3.

Persuasion/argument

A persuasion/argument text is where a claim is made and evidence to support or oppose the claim is presented (Chambliss & Calfee, 1998). Advertisements are persuasion texts. In an advertisement a claim is made and arguments are given to support the claim. Argument texts present facts and opinions both for and against (e.g., argument for building motorways; building an inland port). Figure 7.14 shows a simple way to present the argument structure.

Figure 7.14. An argument pattern

For	Against

Creating mental images

Creating a mental image of the text being read (or being able to visualise how texts are structured) enhances comprehension (Pressley, 2002). Good readers can see the ribs and bones of the text, the structure: "structure is the key to comprehension—to comprehend a passage is to create a mental structure" (Calfee & Associates, 1984, p. 82). When learning about text structures, it is particularly helpful for students to see (visualise) how the text is structured, and this involves diagramming the text. Diagrams help students to visualise the structure.

For some texts, students can also visualise content. If the child is reading a story set in the countryside, they can create a mental image of pastures and farm animals. If the story is about a dog, they can create a visual image of a dog.

Summarising

Summarising involves teaching how to find the main ideas in texts. To most of us a summary involves being brief and concise, giving the main points, putting it in a nutshell. Research shows that being able to summarise a text enhances comprehension. Block and Pressley (2003, p. 117) define summarising as "the ability to delete irrelevant details, combine similar ideas, condense main ideas, and connect major themes into concise statements that capture the purpose of a reading for the reader." Summarising is embedded within text structure awareness (the third Hi 5! strategy). After the reader has identified the text structure the writer has used, they create a diagram of the structure. Redundant information is discarded, leaving the key ideas. The diagram helps the reader to summarise the main idea/s either orally, visually or in writing (Dymock & Nicholson, 2010).

Vocabulary strategies

In this section we provide a brief overview of how to enhance vocabulary. For a more comprehensive account of teaching vocabulary, refer to *Teaching Vocabulary* (Nicholson & Dymock, 2010).

In a broad sense there are two ways to enhance vocabulary. One is through extensive reading, or print exposure, and the other is through vocabulary strategy instruction. For the student with dyslexia, extensive 'on their own' reading is likely to be a challenge. There are a number of ways around this. Students can be provided with access to audio books, some school journal material is available on CD, and many tablets and computers have text-to-speech technology.

Structural analysis, or teaching students how to break words into their meaningful parts (or morphemes), is one vocabulary strategy that should be taught. Many words in English have more than one morpheme (unit of meaning), particularly the more complex, Latin-based words. At the Anglo-Saxon layer of English this often means breaking compound words into two parts, so *bedroom* is *bed + room*; *skateboard* is *skate – board*; *basketball* is *basket + ball*. Older students should be taught how to break Latin-based words into morphemes. (e.g., *con+struc+tion* in *construction*; or *dis+rupt* in *disrupt*). Knowing the meaning of the morphemes helps to unlock the meaning of the words.

Concept maps, exploring the meaning of words with multiple meanings (e.g., bank, point, saw, needle), and teaching students to use the dictionary and thesaurus are also ways of helping students increase their vocabulary.

Case studies

CASE STUDY 1: Ryan

We met Ryan when he was 9 years 8 months old. He was a Year 5 student who attended a middle-to-large decile 6 primary school. Ryan's mother was one of the first parents to contact the Hamilton Children's Reading Centre, which offers tuition for children experiencing reading difficulties, when it opened in February 2003. She was very concerned about his lack of progress in reading and spelling.

In order to address Ryan's needs a number of assessments were administered on the first day he attended the Reading Centre. These assessments included determining Ryan's knowledge of and/or ability in:

- letter names (and, later, knowledge of letter sounds) (Clay, 2013; see Appendix 1C)
- phonemic awareness, using the Gough-Kastler-Roper Test of Phonemic Awareness (see Nicholson, 2005a; and Appendix 1D)
- decoding ability using the non-word test the Bryant Test of Basic Decoding Skills (see Nicholson, 2005b and Appendix 1B)
- reading words in isolation using the Burt Word Reading Test (Gilmore et al., 1981) (see Appendix 1A)
- reading accuracy, fluency and comprehension using the Neale Analysis of Reading, 3rd ed., Neale et al., 1999)
- spelling using Schonell (Schonell & Schonell, 1960) and later WRAT-4 (Wilkinson & Robertson, 2006) and Invented Spelling (Tunmer & Chapman, 1995) (see Appendix 1E)
- receptive vocabulary using the Picture Peabody Vocabulary Test-III (Dunn, Dunn, & Dunn, 1997) and later PPVT-IV (Dunn & Dunn, 2007a).
Note: PPVT-III and PPVT-IV are untimed tests of receptive vocabulary. They take about 20 minutes to administer and provide an indication of verbal ability/intelligence. No reading is required. The tester says a word (e.g., *bus*, *fence*, *exercising*, *selecting*, *reptile*) and the child points to one of four pictures that best represents the target word.

The initial assessment results, presented in Table 7.5, illustrate that Ryan was experiencing significant decoding difficulties: Ryan is dyslexic.

Table 7.5: Ryan's initial assessment results

	February 2003 Score
Chronological age	9 years 8 months
Alphabet names (52)	50
Alphabet sounds (52)	Did not assess
Phonemic awareness (42)	27
Bryant Test of Basic Decoding Skills (50)	11
Burt Word Reading Test (raw)	20
Burt Word Reading Test (age)	5.10–6.05
Neale Analysis of Reading—Accuracy (raw)	13
Neale Analysis of Reading—Accuracy (age)	6 years 2 months
Neale Analysis of Reading—Accuracy (stanine)	1
Neale Analysis of Reading—Comprehension (raw)	3
Neale Analysis of Reading—Comprehension (age)	6 years 0 months
Neale Analysis of Reading—Comprehension (stanine)	1
Schonell spelling	5 years 6 months
PPVT-III standard score	128
PPVT-III age	14 years 6 months
PPVT-III percentile	97
PPVT stanine	9

Ryan's score of 27/42 on the phonemic awareness measure showed that he had a good awareness of blending and deletion of initial phonemes (7/7 on both assessments) but had some difficulty with segmenting phonemes (5/7) and substitution of first phoneme (4/7). He experienced difficulty deleting the final phoneme (3/7) and substituting the last phoneme (1/7).

Anglo-Saxon decoding strategies based on the Bryant Test of Basic Decoding Skills

The following figure (Figure 7.15 shows Ryan's results for the Bryant Test of Basic Decoding Skills (Bryant, 1975), administered in February 2003.

Figure 7.15: Initial assessment for Ryan: Bryant Test of Basic Decoding Skills

buf ✓	fute *fat*	cosnuv
cos ✓	yode —	relhime
dit *bit*	bime *dim*	defev
fev —	nepe —	gaction
gac ✓	cabe *cad*	prefute
huz *has*	phune —	uncabeness
jod	cho *cop*	exyoded
kib *kid*	shi *kit*	sanwixable
lek *lock*	whe *where*	bufkibber
maz ✓	thade —	vomazful
nuv *nev*	staw	
pof ✓	plew	
quig *kick*	fler	
rel —	smar	
san ✓	blor	
tup ✓	cleef	11/50
vom ✓	troob	
wix ✓	spail	
yeg —	groy	
zad ✓	groaf	

Ryan Feb. 2003

f: Bryant Test of Basic Decoding Skills. New York: Teachers College ess, 1975

The highlighted strategies in Table 7.6 shows the Anglo-Saxon decoding strategies Ryan needs to learn. The highlighted strategies were taught, one by one, from left to right (e.g., short vowels; long vowels; single consonants, particularly at the end of the word; blends; digraphs).

Table 7.6: The Anglo-Saxon consonants and vowels Ryan needed to learn are highlighted

Anglo-Saxon consonants and vowels Easy to increasing difficulty			
	Consonants		
Single	**Blends**		**Digraphs**
p g d b c v w l r t f j m n s h k q x y z b/d confusion g & b at end of CVC	Initial bl br cl cr dr fl fr gl gr sl pr tr sc sk scr spl sm squ sn str sp st sw tw thr Final - ft -mp -nt -lk		Initial ch sh th wh gh ph Final -ng -ck -ch
	Vowels		
Single			
Short / **Long**	**r & l controlled**		**Digraphs**

a: mad / made
e: pet / Pete
i: Tim / time
o: hop / hope
hops / hopes
hopped / hoped
hopping / hoping
 	
u: cut / cute
	ar: park lard harm
	
	or: for horn short
	
	er: her stern fern
	
	ir: bird thirst sir
	
	ur: fur church burn
	
	al: hall fall call
	     halter falter
	     walk talk
			one sound:
			ai/ay pain, play
			ee meet
			ie piece
			oi/oy foil, toy
			oa boat
			au/aw laud, law
			ew few
			two sounds:
			ea breath, breathe
			ei seize eight
			oo cook food
			ou round soul
			ow cow snow

How can Ryan be helped to overcome his decoding difficulties?

Based on the initial assessment results, the following intervention was established for Ryan. The hour-long, weekly, after-school intervention programme initially focused on developing the following.

Fluency and accuracy

The aim was to develop Ryan's fluency and accuracy when reading connected text.

Phonemic awareness

This covered segmenting, deletion of final phoneme, and substitution of initial and final phonemes.

Word reading

By *word reading* we mean reading basic sight words with speed and accuracy. Word lists such as Edward Fry's or Edward Dolch's can be used. Edward Fry's (2000) list of 200 most common words, in order of frequency, can be found in Appendix 2. There are also a number of websites where teachers can access lists of high-frequency words. Many high-frequency words are non-phonetic, or irregular, and students need to learn these words by sight (e.g., *the*, *any*, *are*, *of*, *off*, *were*, *live*, *they*), because decoding strategies are not helpful here (e.g., decoding strategies will not enable the reader to read *the*).

Ryan progressed to the next list of 25 words when he was able to read the previous list of words with accuracy and speed. Depending on the student, teachers may start with a list of 5 or 10 words (e.g., the first 10 words of list 1 in Appendix 2). Try putting each list of words on coloured paper, laminating it, and cutting it into cards, as shown in Figure 7.16. Each list is assigned a different colour.

Figure 7.16: List words on coloured cards

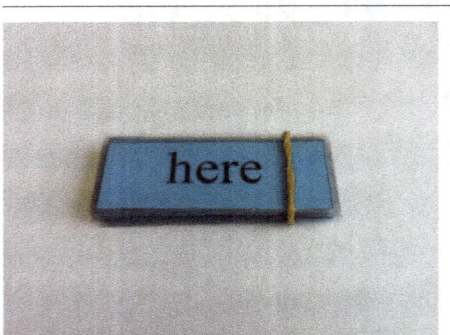 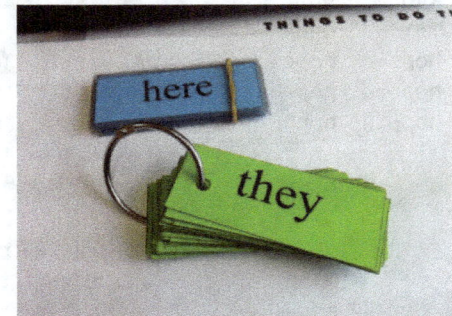

Decoding strategies

Lessons with Ryan involved teaching one decoding strategy at a time. During terms 1 and 2 the main focus was on teaching Ryan the following strategies, primarily using consonant-vowel-consonant (CVC) words:

- short vowel *e* (e.g., *pet, set, jet*; refer to the lesson plan on the short *e* vowel in Appendix 3(a))
- short vowel *u* (e.g., *hut, sun, pup, put*)
- initial consonants *b* and *d* (CVC words)
- initial consonants *y* and *q* (refer to the lesson plan on the consonant y in Appendix 3(b))
- final consonant *g* and *b*
- blends (see highlighted blends in Table 7.6 above) (refer to the lesson plan on the *st* blend in Appendix 3(c))
- moving towards long vowel sounds—teaching one long vowel (silent *e*) per lesson, or possibly over two lessons (refer to Table 7.6 above, and to the lesson plan on the long *i* vowel in Appendix 3(d))
- after teaching about long vowels, teaching about vowel digraphs (refer to the lesson plan on the vowel digraph *oa* in Appendix 3(e))
- knowing about syllables, particularly closed and open syllables, which helps to know how to read words (refer to the lesson plan on closed and open syllables in Appendix 3(f)).

Although ongoing assessment occurs throughout an intervention, formal assessments are administered at the end of the year. The 2003 end-of-year results showed that Ryan was making decoding progress (see Table 7.7). The 2004 end-of-year results show that Ryan's decoding skills continued to develop the following year.

Table 7.7: Assessment results for Ryan: end of first year and following year

	December 2003	February 2004	December 2004
Chronological age	10 years 5 months	10 years 8 months	11 years 5 months
Alphabet names (52)	52	50	52
Alphabet sounds (52)	Did not assess	52	52
Phonemic awareness (42)	42	36	41
Bryant Test of Basic Decoding Skills (50)	32	20	35
Burt Word Reading Test (raw)	29	24	49
Burt Word Reading Test (age)	7.1	6.05	8 years 6 months
Neale Analysis of Reading—Accuracy (raw)	20	10	37
Neale Analysis of Reading—Accuracy (age)	6 years 7 months	6 years 3 months	7 years 10 months
Neale Analysis of Reading—Accuracy (stanine)	1	1	2
Neale Analysis of Reading— Comprehension (raw)	9	4	17
Neale Analysis of Reading— Comprehension (age)	6 years 11 months	6 years 4 months	8 years 5 months
Neale Analysis of Reading— Comprehension (stanine)	1	1	3
Schonell spelling		6 years 8 months	6 years 9 months

Ryan's decoding skills continued to progress and he gained NCEA Levels 1, 2 and 3. Ryan is presently completing a BSc degree majoring in chemistry. Ryan's story is told in this book's companion video *Talking about Dyslexia*. (See www.nzcer.org.nz/nzcerpress/new-zealand-dyslexia-handbook.)

CASE STUDY 2: William, Year 8

William was formally diagnosed with dyslexia in Year 4 (refer to 'William's story' in the video *Talking about Dyslexia*). William, an articulate boy with a large vocabulary, entered school with enthusiasm. His Year 1 and 2 teachers indicated to his parents that he would do well at school and that his reading would soon "take off". By Year 3

William was aware that he was not making age-appropriate progress in reading and spelling. His poor reading and spelling skills were beginning to have an impact on his self-esteem and feelings of self-worth, and his enthusiasm for school was disappearing. After 3 years of schooling William, undoubtedly one of the brightest pupils in the decile 4, 250–300-pupil school, was reading and spelling below age level. The school had few answers for his poor progress. His parents were also at a loss, given that their observations indicated that William was an intelligent boy. It is not unusual for adults to engage in conversation with William on topics ranging from science and finance, to the Bible, history and politics.

William's poor decoding and spelling skills were affecting not only his school work, but his home life as well. William was becoming increasingly unhappy at school, withdrawing from his peers, confused because he knew he should be able to decode and spell but couldn't. At times William was told by his teacher to "try harder" when in fact he tried harder than anyone else in the class. Writing was a slow process for William. At times he had to stay in during play time and lunch time to finish his work. In essence he was being punished for having decoding and spelling difficulties and for 'not trying hard enough'. Even when William thought he had completed the writing task it was not unusual for him to be told that he had "not written enough". Asking William to write another page was like telling him to climb Mt Everest.

During term 1 of Year 4 William's mother went to school to speak to his teacher about his lack of progress in reading and spelling. When she entered his classroom she knew, without asking, that something was amiss. William's body language, among his peers, spoke volumes. Enough was enough: after more than 3 years of schooling with limited reading and spelling progress, William's parents made an appointment with a specialist in order to identify what was preventing him from achieving success in decoding and spelling.

The result of the diagnosis: William is dyslexic.

There was a sense of relief for both William and his parents because they now had an explanation for why he was not making adequate progress in decoding and spelling. The next step was to find help for William. Unfortunately there were limited options. The school was not equipped, funded or knowledgeable enough to provide the necessary tuition. One option was private tuition. Following formal assessment ($500 plus), tuition is typically $40–45 per hour, which is prohibitive for many families. William's parents heard about a reading centre associated with the University of Waikato that provides specialist diagnosis and tuition for children experiencing reading difficulties. A place became available for William at the beginning of his 6th year at school.

Assessment overview

Initial assessments in February 2011 showed that at 10 years 1 month William knew all the letter names but did not know all the sounds each letter represents (see Table 7.8). William's score of 32 on the phonemic awareness measure placed him where a good 6-year-old reader would be (i.e. a reader 4 years below William's chronological age). A 10-year-old reader making age-appropriate progress typically scores between 45 and 50 on the Bryant Test of Decoding Skills; William scored 20, a level where most 7-year-olds would be. William's reading accuracy age, based on standardised measures, placed him between 7.5 years and 8 years 1 month. His spelling age placed him 3 years below his chronological age. William's initial assessment results are reported in Table 7.8.

Table 7.8: William's initial assessment results at the Hamilton Reading Centre

Assessment	February – Assessment 1a
Chronological age	10 years 1 month
Alphabet names (52)	52
Alphabet sounds (52)	39
Phonemic awareness (42)	32
Bryant Test of Basic Decoding Skills (50)	20
Burt Word Reading Test (raw)	44
Burt Word Reading Test (age)	8 years 1 month
Neale Analysis of Reading—Accuracy (raw)	31
Neale Analysis of Reading—Accuracy (age)	7 years 5 months
Neale Analysis of Reading—Accuracy (stanine)	2
Neale Analysis of Reading—Comprehension (raw)	14
Neale Analysis of Reading—Comprehension (age)	7 years 11 months
Neale Analysis of Reading—Comprehension (stanine)	2
Schonell spelling	7 years 3 months
PPVT-IV standard score	132
PPVT-IV age	15 years 9 months
PPVT-IV percentile	98
PPVT-IV stanine	9

William scored 32/42 on the phonemic awareness measures; 7/7 each for deletion of first phoneme, phoneme segmentation and substitution of first phoneme; 3/7 for blending phonemes; 5/7 for deletion of last phoneme; and 3/7 for substitution of first phoneme (see Figure 7.16).

Figure 7.17: Initial assessment for William: phonemic awareness

Chart 1: Gough-Kastler-Roper Phonemic Awareness Test

Teacher Instructions: Remember that this is **not** a reading test. You have to **read aloud** the questions to the child. The test has six subtests. Total of 42 items.

Give the practice item first in each subtest. The answers to each item are given in brackets.

If the child has trouble during the test, give supportive comments like 'Good boy/girl', 'That's good', 'OK, let's try another one'. You can give explanations for the practice test items.

1. Blending
Practice: "Say c-a-t. What word is c-a-t?" (answer = cat)
- n-i-ce (nice) ✓
- t-oo (too) ✓
- h-e (he) ✓
- r-a-ke (rake) *tek.*
- t-r-ai-n (train) *tain.*
- p-l-a-ne (plane) *playin*
- f-u-nn-y (funny) *fin ee.* 3

2. Deletion of first phoneme
Practice: 'Say cat. Now say cat without the k.' (answer = at)
- top (t) (op) ✓
- gasp (g) (asp) ✓
- find (f) (ind) ✓
- paint (p) (aint) ✓
- up (u) (p) ✓
- at (a) (t) ✓
- so (s) (o) ✓   7

3. Deletion of last phoneme
Practice: 'Say cat. Now say cat without the t.' (answer = ca)
- same (m) (sa) *sum.*
- me (e) (m) *made no sound.*
- ate (t) (a) ✓
- go (o) (g) ✓
- frog (g) (fro) ✓
- grab (b) (gra) ✓
- stride (d) (stri) ✓   5

4. Phonemic segmentation
Practice: 'Say cat. What are the three sounds in cat?' (answer = ceh-ah-teh)
- 2 no (n-o) ✓
- 2 at (a-t) ✓
- 2 up (u-p) ✓
- 3 keep (k-ee-p) ✓
- 3 man (m-a-n) ✓
- 3 teeth (t-ee-th) ✓
- 4 into (i-n-t-o) *to* ✓   7.

5. Substitution of first phoneme
Practice: 'Say cat. Now, instead of k, start the new word with f.' (answer = fat)
- ball   b   c   (call) ✓
- goat   g   b   (boat) ✓
- took   t   c   (cook) ✓
- fish   f   d   (dish) ✓
- two   t   z   (zoo) ✓
- chair ch p   (pair) ✓
- meat   m   f   (feat) ✓   7.

6. Substitution of last phoneme
Practice: 'Say cat. Instead of t, end the new word with p.' (answer = cap)
- park   k   t   (part) ✓
- run   n   g   (rug) ✓
- late   t   m   (lame) *limb*
- mess   s   n   (men) *mens.*
- rope   p   d   (rode) ✓
- fame   m   s   (face) —
- wet   t   b   (web) *bet.* 3

Total Score = 32/42

Interpreting scores
There are no New Zealand norms for this test, but the following scores are a guide:
- five-year-olds (beginning of year):   low pre-reading = 5;   high pre-reading = 10
- five-year-olds (end of year):   poorer readers = 10;   better readers = 25
- six-year-olds (end of year):   poorer readers = 25;   better readers = 35

Copyright acknowledgement: Reprinted with permission of P.B. Gough. Instructions adapted by Tom Nicholson. Source: Roper (1984).

Anglo-Saxon decoding strategies based on the Bryant Test of Basic Decoding Skills

Figure 7.18 shows William's results for the Bryant Test of Basic Decoding Skills (Bryant, 1975). The highlighted strategies in Table 7.9 shows the Anglo-Saxon decoding strategies William needs to learn. The highlighted strategies were taught, one by one, from left to right (e.g., short vowels; long vowels; single consonants, particularly at the end of the word; blends; digraphs).

Initial consonant f

Figure 7.18: Initial assessment for William: Bryant Test of Basic Decoding Skills

BRYANT TEST OF BASIC DECODING SKILLS

Tester instructions: Score as correct if the pupil pronounces the made-up words as shown below. Write down the error if the pupil makes a mistake (e.g., reads "buf" as "but"). Be sure to explain to the pupil that these are not real words. They are the names of children from another planet, and they speak a different language to us. Stop testing after 10 consecutive errors. Ask the pupil to look at the rest of the words and to read out any words that can be decoded. Then score out of 50.

1. buf (as in "muff")	✓	26. phune (as in "tune")	fiu ^
2. cos (as in "toss")	✓	27. cho (as in "go")	✓
3. dit (as in "hit")	^ drit ✗	28. shi (as in "shy")	✓
4. fev (as in "Bev")	vet ^	29. whe (as in "he")	✓
5. gac (as in "sack")	grat ^	30. thade (as in "made")	✗ ^
6. huz (as in "buzz")	hauzat ^	31. staw (as in "store")	✓
7. jod (as in "cod")	✓	32. plew (as in "flew")	pew
8. kib (as in "rib")	✓	33. fler (as in "her")	
9. lek (as in "neck"	linbi ^	34. smar (as in "bar")	sam reversal.
10. maz (as in "jazz")	maze ^	35. blor (as in "floor")	board ^
11. nuv (as in "love")	nanz ^	36. cleef (as in "leaf")	cleeth ^
12. pof (as in "off")	✓	37. troob (as in "tube")	✓
13. quig (as in "big")	✓	38. spail (as in "mail")	✓
14. rel (as in "bell")	rul ^	39. groy (as in "boy")	✓
15. san (as in "pan")	✓	40. groaf (as in "loaf")	grif
16. tup (as in "cup")	tran ^	41. cosnuv (as in cos-nuv)	cosnuve
17. vom (as in "from")	✓	42. relhime (as in rel-hime)	re hine
18. wix (as in "six")	✓	43. defev (as in de-fev)	dufue
19. yeg (as in "leg")	✓	44. gaction (as in gak-shun)	raction
20. zad (as in "bad")	✓	45. prefute (as in pre-fute)	perfom
21. fute (as in "cute")	^	46. uncabeness (as in un-cabe-ness)	
22. yode (as in "code")	yowd ^	47. exyoded (as in ex-yode-ed)	
23. bime (as in "time")	✓	48. sanwixable (as in san-wicks-able)	
24. nepe (as in "keep")	✓	49. bufkibber (as in buff-kibb-er)	
25. cabe (as in "babe")	crab ^	50. vomazful (as in vom-az-ful)	

Reference: Bryant, D. (1975). *Bryant Test of Basic Decoding Skills*. Unpublished manuscript, Teachers College, Columbia University, New York

20/50.

Chapter 7: Teaching children with dyslexia to read

Table 7.9: The Anglo-Saxon consonants and vowels William needed to learn are highlighted

Consonants		
Single	**Blends**	**Digraphs**
Initial consonant **f** End consonant only **p** g d b **c** v w l r **t** f j m n s h **k** q x y **z**	Initial **bl** br cl cr dr **fl** fr gl gr sl **pl** pr tr sc sk scr spl **sm** squ sn str sp st sw tw thr Final -ft -mp -nt -lk	Initial ch sh **th** wh gh ph Final -ng -ck -ch
	Vowels	
Single		
Short Long	**r & l controlled**	**Digraphs**

a: mad **made**
e: **pet** **Pete**
i: Tim **time**
o: hop **hope**
  hops hopes
  hopped hoped
  hopping hoping
 	
u: **cut** **cute**
	ar: park lard harm
	
	or: for horn short
	
	er: her stern fern
	
	ir: bird thirst sir
	
	ur: fur church burn
	
	al: hall fall call
	  halter falter
	  walk talk
		one sound:
		  ai/ay pain, play
		  ee meet
		  ie piece
		  oi/oy foil, toy
		  oa boat
		  au/aw taut, law
		  eu/ew feud, few
		two sounds:
		  ea breath, breathe
		  ei seize eight
		  oo cook food
		  ou round soul
		  ow cow snow

William received one-to-one tuition at the after-school Hamilton Children's Reading Centre for 1 hour, once a week, during the school term. The primary focus of the intervention was on increasing William's phonemic awareness and on teaching decoding strategies. William also practised reading words in context and words in isolation.

The December end-of-year results showed that William had made good gains (see Table 7.10), but stanine scores for decoding remained below average. The comprehension stanine score was low to average. The reason for the low-to-average reading comprehension score was his decoding difficulties.

Table 7.10: William's beginning and end-of-year assessment results for first year at Reading Centre

	February Assessment 1a	December Assessment 1b
Chronological age	10 years 1 month	10 years 10 months
Alphabet names (52)	52	52
Alphabet sounds (52)	39	51
Phonemic awareness (42)	32	39
Bryant Test of Basic Decoding Skills (50)	20	32
Burt Word Reading Test (raw)	44	64
Burt Word Reading Test (age)	8 years 1 month	10 years 3 months
Neale Analysis of Reading—Accuracy (raw)	31	52
Neale Analysis of Reading—Accuracy (age)	7 years 5 months	9 years 4 months
Neale Analysis of Reading—Accuracy (stanine)	2	3
Neale Analysis of Reading—Comprehension (raw)	14	31
Neale Analysis of Reading—Comprehension (age)	7 years 11 months	13 years
Neale Analysis of Reading—Comprehension (stanine)	2	4
Schonell spelling	7 years 3 months	7 years 5 months
PPVT-IV standard score	132	
PPVT-IV age	15.9	
PPVT-IV percentile	98	
PPVT-IV stanine	9	

Table 7.11 shows William's assessment results for his 2nd year at the Hamilton Children's Reading Centre. William's decoding skills continued to progress, and he was now able to decode age-appropriate text, and beyond, although he did so with effort.

Table 7.11: William's 2nd-year assessment results at the Hamilton Reading Centre

	February Assessment 2a	December Assessment 2b
Chronological age	11 years 2 months	11 years 10 months
Alphabet names (52)	52	52
Alphabet sounds (52)	49	45
Phonemic awareness (42)	37	42
Bryant Test of Basic Decoding Skills (50)	32	37
Burt Word Reading Test (raw)	53	76
Burt Word Reading Test (age)	8 years 11 months	11 years 10 months
Neale Analysis of Reading—Accuracy (raw)	52	84
Neale Analysis of Reading—Accuracy (age)	8 years 11 months	13 years+
Neale Analysis of Reading—Accuracy (stanine)	3	5
Neale Analysis of Reading—Comprehension (raw)	25	42
Neale Analysis of Reading— Comprehension (age)	10 years 4 months	13 years +
Neale Analysis of Reading— Comprehension (stanine)	3	9
Schonell (spelling)	7.3 years	8.2
PPVT-IV standard score	143	
PPVT-IV age	Adult	
PPVT-IV percentile	99.9	
PPVT-IV stanine	9	

CASE STUDY 3: Jade, *17 years*

Jade left school in 2011 at the age of 16 without any formal qualifications (i.e. he did not achieve NCEA Levels 1, 2 or 3). Jade has dyslexia, and not one of the three schools he attended (primary, intermediate or high school) addressed his reading needs. After leaving high school Jade started a trades course and specialist tutoring in reading and writing. He does want to achieve. He wants to become a plumber, or possibly join the navy. Since he commenced specialist tutoring he has achieved NCEA Levels 1 and 2.

A number of assessments were administered by his reading tutor so that his reading needs could be addressed (see Tables 7.12 and 7.13).

Table 7.12: Jade's initial assessments results, April 2012

	Assessment
Chronological age	17 years
Alphabet names (52)	52
Alphabet sounds (52)	0 (although Bryant measure below indicated he knew some alphabet sounds)
Phonemic awareness (42)	16
Bryant Test of Basic Decoding Skills (50)	26
Assessment Tool—Reading Comprehension*	Step 2 (about 8–9 years)
Assessment Tool—Vocabulary (emerging, expanding, or extended)	Extended

* Tertiary Education Commission Literacy and Numeracy for Adults—Assessment Tool

Table 7.13: Jade's strengths, areas needing support and implications for the tutor

Jade's strengths	Areas needing support	Challenges Jade will encounter in his coursework	Implications for the tutor
Good vocabulary	Decoding	Unable to comprehend written text if required to decode it	• Arrange print-to-speech software • Read text aloud • Provide more time • Build background knowledge to increase ability to decode content-specific words • Consider readability of text
Keen to learn	Spelling	Difficulty writing due to spelling	• Speech-to-text software • Provide note-taker • Provide more time • Reduce word limit • Offer alternatives to writing to demonstrate understanding • Be sensitive if requiring student to copy large amounts of text

When Jade commenced his reading and spelling tutoring in May 2012 he was reading around the 8–9-year-old level. Jade knew the names of the letters but not the sounds they represented. He had little phonemic awareness and, according to his tutor, he found this assessment "really hard". After a year of tuition (1 hour each week) his tutor wrote,

"His reading has greatly improved, but we still need to work on spelling and writing, which is what we are focusing on at present." The tutor continued:

> He responded really well to the phonological awareness training. I have been working on reading comprehension, decoding, spelling, and writing. I thought we would finish our sessions in December, but he contacted me a few weeks ago saying he wanted to come back. He is a lovely young man and I enjoy teaching him.

The following is a more detailed analysis of the Gough-Kastler-Roper phonemic awareness measure Jade completed as part of his initial assessments (see Nicholson, 2005a):

- blending: 4/7
- deletion of first phoneme: 3/7
- deletion of last phoneme: 3/7
- phoneme segmentation: 0/7
- substitution of first phoneme: 3/7
- substitution of last phoneme: 3/7.

Jade also experienced difficulty with rhyme (e.g., he was unable to complete the sequence *cat, mat, fat* ___; or *rain, pain, plain* ____), or identify the word that does not rhyme (e.g., *sack, back, bite, Jack*): Jade identified *back* as the word that does not rhyme, instead of *bite*.

The results of the Bryant Test of Basic Decoding skills showed that Jade was able to read most consonant-vowel-consonant (CVC) non-words (i.e. 16/20). However he made the following errors:

- *gac* was read as *gaze*
- *nuv* was read as *vin*
- *pof* was read as *pif*
- *yeg*—no attempt was made.

Jade was unable to read words with long vowels *o, i, e,* and *a*, but was able to read words with long *u* vowel sounds. Jade also had difficulty reading r-controlled vowels (*ar, or, er, ir* and *ur*) and vowel digraphs (*oo, ai,* and *oa*). Multi-syllable words also presented a challenge for Jade: he was able to correctly read only 2/10 multisyllabic words in the Bryant Test of Basic Decoding Skills.

The assessment results show that Jade needed to develop his awareness of rhyme and phonemes. There are many Anglo-Saxon decoding strategies he needed to learn before he could move to the more advanced layers of English: Latin and Greek. Table 7.14 highlights the Anglo-Saxon decoding strategies Jade needed to learn.

Table 7.14: The Anglo-Saxon consonants and vowels Jade needed to learn are highlighted

Anglo-Saxon consonants and vowels		
Easy to increasing difficulty		

Consonants		
Single	Blends	Digraphs
p g d b c v w l r t f j m n s h k q x y z	Initial bl br cl cr dr fl fr gl gr sl pr tr sc sk scr spl sm squ sn str sp st sw tw thr Final - ft -mp -nt -lk	Initial **ch** sh th wh gh ph Final -ng -ck -ch
Vowels		
Single		

Short	Long	r & l controlled	Digraphs

a: mad **made**
e: pet **Pete**
i: Tim **time**
o: hop **hope**
   hops hopes
   hopped hoped
   hopping hoping
u: cut cute
		ar: park lard harm
		
		or: for horn short
		
		er: her stern fern
		
		ir: bird thirst sir
		
		ur: fur church burn
		
		al: hall fall call
		    halter falter
		    walk talk
			one sound:
			ai/ay pain, play
			ee meet
			ie piece
			oi/oy foil, toy
			oa boat
			au/aw laud, law
			eu/ew feud, few
			two sounds:
			ea breath, breathe
			ei seize eight
			oo cook food
			ou round soul
			ow cow snow

Jade's tutor began by reviewing short vowels. She then taught Jade each long vowel and the silent *e* rule. Next she progressed to vowel digraphs and r- and l-controlled vowels. Over time Jade's tutor moved to the Latin layer of English, where she taught word analysis strategies (Latin prefixes, roots and suffixes). Jade's tutor wrote, "He picked up decoding skills quickly and his fluency was pretty good." She continued, "So we focused mainly on writing and spelling strategies. The main thing we had to work on was his confidence."

Since receiving the research-based tuition that addressed his decoding needs, Jade has won a permanent position with an Australasian company. He was doing some temping for the company prior to his permanent appointment, but the company was so impressed with his work ethic and skills that when a job came up they asked him to apply. His work now takes him around New Zealand and potentially overseas. While he is still keen to do an apprenticeship one day, he is enjoying the challenge, support and opportunities the company offers.

In these case studies we have discussed the reading needs of three students with dyslexia. We hope the case studies have illustrated the importance of administering appropriate assessments so that the students' reading needs are addressed. Time is not on the side of the student with dyslexia. By the time they are diagnosed with dyslexia and an appropriate intervention programme is put in place, there is typically a large gap between their reading and chronological ages. When we met Ryan he was reading close to 4 years below his chronological reading age. William was reading over 3 years below his chronological age before intervention, and Jade was reading 8 to 9 years below his chronological age. These gaps take time to close.

The following checklist is a useful guide if a student in your class has been formally diagnosed with dyslexia, or has been screened as a possible dyslexic. The checklist would address decoding issues.

Checklist if dyslexia is suspected

or suspects a child has dyslexia, they should administer assessments that answer the following questions:

1. Does the student have phonemic awareness? To what extent?
2. Does the student know the alphabet names?
3. Does the student know the sounds each letter represents?
4. What Anglo-Saxon decoding strategies does the student know?
5. What Anglo-Saxon decoding strategies does the student need to learn?

If the student has a reading age of 9–10 or above:

6. Does the student have the necessary decoding or word analysis strategies for reading multi-syllable Latin based words? (e.g., deconstruction, hospitality)
7. Does the student have the necessary decoding or word analysis strategies for reading Greek based words? (e.g., philosophy, psychology)

Summary

Teaching dyslexic students to read is complex. It requires considerable teacher knowledge and commitment, and the belief that the student will indeed learn to read. Primary and secondary school students with dyslexia typically have decoding difficulties. It is likely that reading comprehension will be good once dyslexic students develop age-appropriate decoding strategies. This has certainly been the case for Ryan and William. In fact their reading comprehension has now surpassed their chronological age. Given their PPVT scores, this was to be expected. Teachers must also be aware that vocabulary and reading comprehension may be affected, particularly for older readers (e.g., high school students) who have been unable to read due to decoding difficulties. If this is the case, students will need to be taught vocabulary and comprehension strategies in addition to decoding strategies.

CHAPTER 8

Teaching pupils with dyslexia to spell and write

Introduction

The chapter will cover four things. First, it will explain the spelling process and what it involves for the dyslexic pupil. Second, it will explain what spelling skills the teacher has to develop in their pupils. Third, it gives specific teaching strategies to encourage better spelling. Fourth, it explains that writing for the dyslexic pupil may be difficult because they have trouble organising their ideas. The writing section gives examples of how the dyslexic writer can present their ideas in an organised fashion whether it is a narrative story or an informational or persuasive text. Appendices at the end of the book give spelling exercises related to this chapter, including a spelling programme.

Part 1: Spelling

How do our teachers teach spelling?

A random sample survey of 405 New Zealand teachers (McNeill & Kirk, 2014) found that most teachers did not teach their pupils how to spell phonologically, that is, did not teach sound-letter relationships, phonological awareness, or spelling patterns even though more than 90 percent of teachers said that it was important to teach these things. The reason for this could be lack of training in teaching spelling.

Nearly seven in 10 teachers said they did not receive enough preparation in their teacher training to teach spelling. They said that their most common problem in teaching spelling was a lack of time.

More than 8 in 10 teachers said they assessed spelling. Seven in 10 teachers said they used a commercial spelling programme to teach spelling. The strategies teachers most used when putting together spelling lists for teaching was to include high frequency words (61percent) and common spelling patterns (51percent).

More than half of teachers asked pupils to learn lists of high-frequency words or words with common spelling patterns. Using lists is also common in classrooms in the US, where every Monday pupils are given a list of words to learn during the week and they are tested on Friday (Hilden & Jones, 2012).

In a smaller study of staff in one school, Morris (2012) found that nearly all the staff taught spelling as part of their regular classroom programme (26 out of 28) though half the staff reported they lacked confidence about teaching spelling (12 out of 23) and grammar (12 out of 24). The survey found that nearly all teachers valued spelling accuracy (18 out of 21).

Strategies mentioned for helping pupils to spell words were: sound it out (e.g., say first sound, write, say middle sound, write, say last sound, write), use the dictionary, break word into syllables, say word slowly and spell out the sounds, think of a word that rhymes with the word, over-line it and come back to it later. Teachers spent from 10–25 minutes a day on spelling. They used weekly spelling lists for pupils to learn. A common strategy recommended to pupils for learning to spell words was: look-cover-write-check.

The dyslexic speller

Not everyone is a poor speller, but many students with dyslexia have this as their biggest issue. Dyslexia and spelling difficulties go hand in hand. The pupil with dyslexia is likely to have good ideas for writing but to have trouble putting them on paper because of poor spelling. We know from the simple view of writing that the competent writer is a good speller and has good ideas as well. Given that the main difference between the good writer and the writer with dyslexia is a difference in spelling ability, the teacher will make more impact on the dyslexic pupil's writing by attending to spelling rather than to ideas. But how do you improve their spelling?

Yes, we would like students with dyslexia to spell well, but they don't have to spell well straight away. The aim is to have them spell phonologically with invented spellings so that at least you can read their writing. We need to teach the dyslexic pupil to spell according to the sounds of words, and this means teaching them how to split up words, phoneme by phoneme, and spell that way. For example, it would be better to spell *home* as *hom* or *have* as *hav* or *school* as *skuel*, which are fairly understandable. Teaching invented spelling helps pupils to get off to a better start (Ouellette & Sénéchal, 2008; Ouellette, Sénéchal, & Haley, 2013; Sénéchal, Ouellette, Pagan, & Lever, 2011).

What is spelling?

Spelling involves writing alphabetic characters in a sequence that corresponds to the sequence of phonemes in spoken words and also matches conventional spelling as revealed in a dictionary. In English, learning to spell even common words is difficult because the same sound can have more than one spelling (e.g., the /oo/ sound in *boot* and *soup* and *crew*). The same letter can represent more than one sound (e.g., *c* in *coffee* and *c* in *cigar*). Some sounds are spelled differently to normal (e.g., *ph* in *phone*). Some letters are silent (e.g., the *e* in *house*). English spelling is complex, but it is also systematic, which is something that we need to explain to students with dyslexia so that they can see that there is method and not madness.

Phases in learning to spell

Ehri (2005) found that pupils learning to spell (and read) go through a series of phases. The first phase is pre-alphabetic, where the student does not know the letters and sounds and so they invent them. The second phase is the important one for invented spelling: the student knows the names and sounds of letters, and has some phonemic awareness, but they are not able to spell unfamiliar words completely. They are able to invent spellings using their letter–name knowledge; for example, YL (for *while*) and MFN (for *muffin*).

Gentry (2000) suggests five phases:
1. **random**, where the student uses letters but they are strung together in a random way (e.g., 'XRIAYETSIMCK', for 'I am going to the shop')
2. **semi-phonemic**, where the pupil can represent some of the sounds in words (e.g., 'I w f a wk' for 'I went for a walk')
3. **phonemic**, where the pupil spells words strictly according to their sounds—this is called 'invented' or 'temporary' spelling (e.g., 'I LIK SCOOL' for 'I like school'

or 'Wen skl was finised I wnt to the libee my mm sed to me haree up and I fwnd sum bks' (When school was finished I went to the library. Mum said to me hurry up and I found some books)
4. **transitional**, where the student shows some knowledge of conventional spellings but they are not used correctly as yet (e.g., spells *cake* as *caek*. The miscue shows that the pupil is aware of the conventional spelling where "cake" has the silent e at the end of the word.
5. **conventional**, where the student spells correctly.

Figure 8.1: Summary of the developmental steps in learning to spell

Developmental steps in spelling cake				
bfg	kc	cak	caek	cake
Random	Semi-phonemic	Phonemic	Transitional	Conventional

The beginnings of spelling

Cue spelling

Gough et al. (1992) found that children's early attempts at spelling did not follow the sound pattern of words, but their memory of the 'look' of the word. They call it 'cue' spelling. The problem is that in remembering words by their overall look, pupils are likely to spell the wrong words (e.g., spell *rain* as *yes*, or spell *with* as *play*.

Cue spellers rely on ineffective strategies. They are not using phonological recoding skills. Instead, they rely on their memory of the look of the word, or on one or two distinctive cues, or on the first letter but the rest of the word is a jumble of letters. These students have not understood the alphabetic principle that letters represent the phonemes that are in spoken words.

Cue spelling	Spelling words by a distinctive cue, e.g., spelling 'rain' as 'rup' because they remembered the 'r'—or even writing a different word altogether.

Cypher spelling

Gough et al. (1992) explained that invented spelling is the next stage after cue spelling. It shows understanding of the 'cipher'. If a student uses cipher spelling, the pupil must understand the alphabetic principle. This requires phonemic awareness; that is, knowledge that spoken words can be segmented into their component phonemes, as in *u-p* or *t-ee-th*, and that these phonemes map onto the alphabet.

Cipher spelling	Knowledge of how to spell regular words like *fish* and *cat*, or when the beginner spells *woz* for *was*.

The cipher is the way the phonemes map onto letters, and enables the beginning speller to spell many words correctly because their spellings are regular (Gough & Hillinger, 1980). The limitation of cipher spelling (Gough et al., 1992) is that it only works for regularly spelled words.

Limitations of cipher spelling

Cipher spelling does not work so well for irregularly spelled words like *yacht*, misspelled as *yot*, or *was*, misspelled as *woz*. It also does not work so well for words that are polygraphic (spelled in more than one way); for example, there are two spellings of the /ee/ sound, so that the pupil might spell *green* or *grean*.

Irregular spellings: how do we learn them?

Learning irregular spellings, called 'lexical' spellings, requires the student to memorise the parts that are unusual. The question, though, is whether this has to be done as a total visual memorisation or whether the pupil only needs to remember the part that is irregular (e.g., the *ach* in *yacht*, or the *a* in *was*.

Lexical spelling	Knowledge of the correct spellings to use (e.g., is the /e/ in *green* spelled *ee* or *ea*?).

Gough and Walsh (1991) found that the ability to spell irregular words depends on knowledge of the cipher; that is, knowledge of regular letter–sound rules. They found that pupils who have good cipher knowledge (i.e., can read and spell regular words) are better at learning to read and spell exception words. Ehri (2005) also argues this point: once children are able to read and spell phonemically, they are able to move to a consolidated phase in learning whereby the exact letters of words are stored in memory as sight words.

Invented spelling

Invented spelling	This is where the names of letters are used to spell the phonemes in words inventively, as in *GRF* for *giraffe*, *MFN* for *muffin*, *RUF* for *rough*, *VEGTIBL* for *vegetable*.

Evidence for cipher spelling, that is, spelling according to the phonemes in words, comes from research on invented spelling. An example of a sentence containing invented spelling is: "If I woz a dog I wood chas stiks and pla al dae" (If I was a dog I would chase sticks and play all day).

Read (1971) discovered preschool children who invented their own spellings using letter names to represent phonemes in words. Treiman (1993, 1994) found further support for invented spelling when she studied the 6,000 spellings made by 43 Year 1 pupils over a year. Read's and Treiman's research have revolutionised our understanding of how children learn to spell (Read & Treiman, 2013).

Teaching to spell Anglo-Saxon, Romance (Latin and French) words and Greek words

Anglo-Saxon words

See the summary in Figure 8.2. These spelling patterns are described in Chapter 7. The basic CVC pattern is the easiest. Calfee and Patrick (1995) explain that with just three consonants (*p, t, k*) and one vowel (*a*) you can make nine CVC patterns even if they are not all real words: *at, ap, ak, pat, pak, tap, tak, kap, kat*. Anglo-Saxon words are not very long, usually two syllables. New words are made up as compound words. There are a few prefixes and suffixes, not many.

Romance words

See Figure 8.2. The letter-sound patterns make use of morphology. Prefixes and suffixes have meaning. The "ti" pattern in words like "disruption" has a /sh/ sound. Words ending in "ian" mean someone who does something, e.g., magician, physician. Words are longer, can be three or more syllables.

Greek words

See Figure 8.2. The letter-sound patterns are similar to Anglo-Saxon. They do not use prefixes and suffixes. Multi-syllable words are like compound words but each part is not necessarily a real word, e.g., agora-phobia (fear of public places), thermo-meter (measure of heat), monochrome (one colour).

Figure 8.2: Summary of the spelling patterns for Anglo-Saxon, Romance, and Greek words (Calfee et al., 1984)

	Elements of English spelling		
	Letter–sound patterns	Syllable patterns	Morpheme patterns
Anglo Saxon	cap stand that pin/pine car beat	tennis sister napkin hundred	railroad pigtails like/unlike/likely
Romance	direction spatial excellent	inter- intro- -ity	prediction disrupt ve admission
Greek	physics chemist	auto- micro-	microscope chronometer physiology

Learning about morphology—meaningful units of words

From the age of 7 onwards pupils can benefit from learning about prefixes and suffixes and root words, in other words, morphology (Hurry et al., 2005). Prefixes are meaningful units at the start of words, e.g., *re-* to mean again, as in *re-open* and *re-write*. Suffixes are at the end of words to indicate things like part of speech or tense or plurality, e.g., adding *s* to the ends of words to indicate the plural form, as in *cats*, *dogs*, or *-ed*, to indicate the past tense.

Children intuitively use morphology when deciding how to spell the endings of words that use *s* as a suffix (Bryant, 2002). The rule is that if it is a plural of the word, then we spell *s* even if the sound is either /s/, as in *cats*, or /z/ as in *dogs*. If the ending of the noun is possessive, as in *the boy's bag*, then we add an apostrophe before the *s* (*'s*). If the noun is plural then the apostrophe is after the *s* (e.g., the boys' bags). The student also learns intuitively that if the word ends in /ks/ then we use *s* if it is a plural (e.g., *socks*) or possessive (e.g., *the sock's colour is red*), but if the /ks/ is not one of these endings then we use *x*, or sometimes *xe* (e.g., fox, axe, fix).

Children at first come up with a general rule; for example, that *-ed* is for the past tense of regular verbs (e.g., *covered*, *jumped*), and then overgeneralise the rule to irregular verbs (e.g., *sleped* for *slept*, *keped* for *kept*) but eventually they realise there are exceptions to the general rule and work out the exact rule. For the poor speller, though, the correct form of the rule is not intuitively obvious and it will help if the teacher explains it (Bryant, Nunes, & Snaith, 2000; Bryant, 2002).

Suggested spelling strategies

1. Teaching beginning sounds (Borgia & Owles, 2011). You need:
   - Small whiteboard, marker pen
   - Alphabet chart on view
   - Put pupils in teams of four
   - Select words from the Big Book, say the word, pupils write the letter to go with the first sound of the word
   - Pupils can collaborate check what they have written on their whiteboards
   - Teacher pulls number out of hat, e.g., team 3—pupils in that team give their answer, hold up whiteboards

2. Use sound boxes (Clay, 1993; Joseph, 1999)
   - Select word from Big Book, e.g., "train"
   - Pupils draw a sound box, one box for each phoneme

   - Pupils listen for the first sound, write it, and so on

t	r	ai	n

   - Teacher asks them to point to each sound as she says it, t-r-ai-n

3. Turtle talk (Gough & Lee, 2007; Tse & Nicholson, 2014)
   - Teacher selects some words from the Big Book that illustrate a spelling rule, e.g., "rain", "say", "cake"
   - Teacher writes the words on the whiteboard, underlines the phonemes, as in "r ai n"
   - Teacher says the word slowly as in Turtle Talk and points to each letter while saying that phoneme
   - Pupils read along with the teacher
   - Teacher explains that for the "ai" sound we spell "ai" in the middle of the word and "ay" at the end. For "cake", the "ay" sound is signalled by the silent e
   - Pupils read the words again, phoneme by phoneme

4. Morpheme boxes (Borgia & Owles, 2011)
   - Choose difficult word from Big Book, e.g., "retrospect"
   - Divide word into prefix and root word: retro/spect
   - Discuss meaning of "retro" (back) and "spect" (see or look)
   - "Retrospect" means to look back

Chapter 8: Teaching pupils with dyslexia to spell and write

5. Word detectives (Johnston, 2013)
    - Discuss with class why words are spelled in unusual ways
    - Example: why is there a silent *e* at the end of "prince"?
    - Reason is that it signals the soft sound /s/ of *c* in words like "dance". It also signifies the soft sound /j/ of *g* in words like judge
    - Example: why is there a silent *e* at the end of "give"?
    - Reason: We do not usually end a word with *v* so the printers in the old days added the *e*, as in "love", "have", and so on.

6. Word mapping (Murray & Steinen, 2011)
    - Teach students how to spell words in chunks
    - Problem: Student spells "miscellaneous" as "miscllious"
    - Pronounce the first syllable, "mis", count the phonemes (m-i-s), and spell them
    - Say the second syllable, "cel", count phonemes (c-e-l) and spell
    - Say the third syllable, "la", count phonemes (l-a), spell
    - Count fourth syllable "ne", count phonemes (n-e)
    - Say fifth syllable "ous", count phonemes (ou-s)

7. Teaching the –ed spelling (Snowball, 1993)
    - Select –ed words from Big Book
    - In the children's reader "The King's Birthday" by Dot Meharry, there are lots of –ed words
    - Examples: looked, asked, mixed, ordered, remembered, opened, clapped, cheered, wondered, exploded
    - Explain how –ed is the past tense

8. Hear, spell, read (Ouellette & Tims, 2014)
    - Teacher makes 10 words typed on index cards
    - Pupil has 10 blank cards
    - Pupil reads the word aloud
    - Card shown for 5 seconds, then taken away
    - Pupil spells the word with a pencil or pen
    - If spelling correct, pupil reads it again (if not, correct the spelling)
    - Flip over the card
    - Teacher says word again and pupil spells it
    - Pupil reads the word again

9. Semantic relatives

   Teach students to look for semantic relatives that reveal the correct spelling (e.g., the *e* in comp*e*te helps to spell *competition*, the *ea* in *heal* helps to spell *healthy*). For example, when they are trying to spell a word like *competition*, if they think how they spell its relative *compete*, it will help to avoid errors like *compitition*. Likewise, if they remember how to spell *heal*, they are more likely to spell *healthy* rather than *helthy*. If they think of *medical*, it will help with *medicine* instead of spelling it as *medisin*.

10. Teach mnemonics

    Teach mnemonics such as 'The principal is your pal' and 'There is a lion in battalion'. Crist and Smith (2008) reported that high school students remembered the mm in accommodation by creating a mental image of a money-hungry hotel owner cramming as many people as possible into the hotel's rooms.

    Some students forget to write the *e* in sincere. A mnemonic can be a story to help you remember the spelling. To remind students why there is an *e* at the end of the word, the teacher explained that in Roman times less reputable potters used to cover up the cracks in their pots by coating them with wax. When the customer heated the pots, they broke up. As a result, the reputable potters inscribed "sin" (without) "cere" (wax) on their pots to let the customer know that the pots were not flawed. Students remember the spellings of "sin" and "cere" and this helps them to spell "sincere" correctly.

11. Over-pronounce words

    Spelling is remembered better if pupils over-pronounce words to remind them of the parts that are hard to spell. For example, many pupils write "choclit" for chocolate but if they over-pronounce the word, it helps their spelling, e.g., choc-oh-late (Ehri, 1987). Another example is the irregular word friend which can be over-pronounced as fry-end.

12. Discuss the meanings of words

    Students learn the spellings of words better when they see them, say them, write them, and talk about what they mean (Ehri, 2013).

Phonograms

Appendix 5 has two phonogram charts (Greaney, 2000). Wyllie and Durrell (1970) argued that it was easier to learn to spell vowel sounds if children learned 35 rimes where the sound was predictable and that this would enable them to read/spell 500 words. Chart A has phonograms (or rimes) that have the short vowel sound while

Chart B mostly has rimes with r-affected or long vowel sounds. Kessler and Treiman (2003) suggest using phonograms (or words with rime patterns) to help students spell one-syllable words. They argue that children find it easier to segment words into onsets (the initial consonants of the word) and rimes (the vowel and the consonants after it). Students can find other words that have the rime patterns and students can find the rimes (e.g., *heater* has the *-eat* rime) (Greaney, 2000). Give spelling tests that cover the rime patterns.

Spelling lists

Appendix 6 provides the scope and sequence of a spelling programme a teacher can use with the regular class and with poor spellers. The lists focus on the vowel sounds because they are the most difficult to spell.

Part 2: Teaching writing

Students with dyslexia usually have good ideas but may have trouble organising the ideas into a coherent piece of writing. We will look at some simple strategies for teaching writing.

Kinds of writing

As we saw in Chapter 7, there are three main kinds of writing:
- stories (narrative writing), where you write about real or imagined events using the structure of setting, characters, plot, and theme
- information texts, where you explain some factual information using a structure that is either description (a list, a description of one thing, compare–contrast, or hierarchy) or sequence (step-by-step, cause–effect or problem–solution)
- argument, where you state your position (your claim) and then back it up with ideas in support of the claim.

Teaching narrative writing

Table 8.5: Features that apply to different parts of story structure

Structure	Features of the structure			
Setting	Time	Place	Mood	
Characters	Appearance	Personality	Behaviour	
Plot	Problem	Response	Action	Outcome
Theme				

The plot is the key to a good story. An important point to understand about narrative text is the plot and how it works. This is the foundation for any effective narrative writing. The plot is the heart of the narrative. It is where the action takes place. Novice writers view narratives as having a beginning, middle and end. As authors they want to start at the beginning and continue writing until the narrative ends. This is fine, but they often write a long narrative that lacks structure. It consists of 'and then, and then, and then', as if the narrative is a diary of events.

A plot is more than that. It starts with a problem. Every story has a problem. For example, start with a problem such as 'Our street is turning into a car yard for burglars. Just about every week a car is smashed into or taken.' Then the plot in the story could be about how you see a car thief in the middle of the night and how you solve this problem.

Explain to students that narrative structure includes four components: setting, characters, plot, and theme (Dymock, 2007; Dymock & Nicholson, 2012). A narrative tells the reader who (characters) did what to whom (plot), when and where (setting).

Theme

Narratives usually also have a theme or message, but it is often not explicitly stated. It is important for pupils to think of what the message of the story will be in that this will give a point to the story.

Setting

The setting explains where the narrative takes place, the time it takes place, and the mood of the place. Often pupils give the where but not the time or the mood.

Characters

The characters in a narrative can be major or minor. You can describe their appearance, personality, and behaviour. Characters can play a part in the story or be a narrator of the story. A suggestion is for the pupil to avoid having characters who are narrators because being a narrator means knowing how the story will unfold and this puts a lot of pressure on the pupil as writer. With characters who are not the narrator, you can let the plot unfold through the characters and they do not have to know what will happen next.

Plot

The plot is made up of episodes. Each episode has four parts: a problem, reaction to the problem, action to solve the problem, and outcome or solution. Good stories usually have complications to keep the reader's interest. For example, just as everyone seems happy, introduce a complication so that they are all on red alert again.

An example of a story written by a grade 6 pupil is given in Figure 8.4. It has a title and a good opening that hooks the reader in with its talk of watching cartoons. It seems a happy scene, until there is a fire. The story has a setting, characters, and a plot (problem, action, outcome). There is an unstated theme that we can all survive an extreme situation.

Figure 8.4: "The storm": Students are shown a picture on a stormy day with lightning causing several houses in a suburb to catch fire. They then write a story that fits the picture

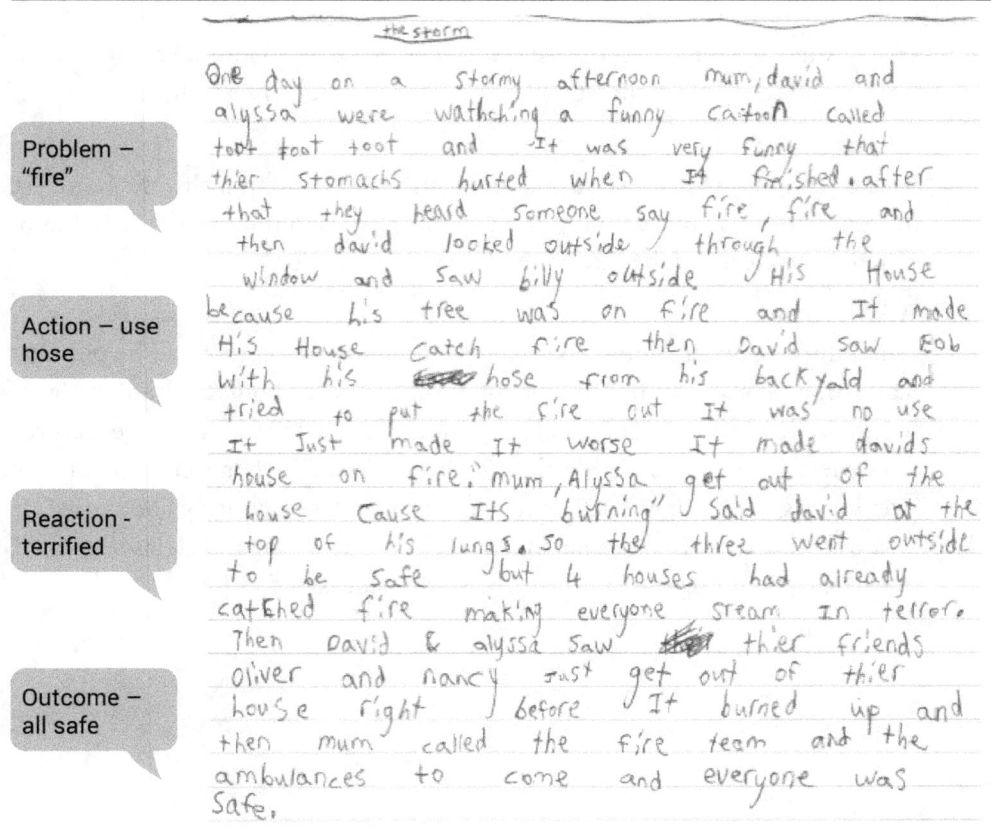

There is a plot with a problem (the fire), reaction (feelings of terror), action (use hose, call the fire engines) and outcome (all safe). It has a sense of excitement. There is dialogue to bring the characters alive. There is a happy ending. It has all the elements of a story and an unstated theme that if we do not panic we can all survive an extreme situation. It has characters (Mum, David, Alyssa, Billy, Bob, Oliver, Nancy) although their characters could be developed with more description of their feelings and appearance. The ending seems rushed: it does not explain what happened when the fire engines arrived. In terms of conventions, it lacks paragraph structure and there are spelling mistakes here and there, but overall it is a good attempt.

Teaching informational writing

Explain to students that factual writing is not like narrative writing. It has a different set of structures. There are three main kinds of factual text: descriptive, sequential and persuasive (Dymock & Nicholson, 2007, 2012; Ministry of Education, 1996).

1. Descriptive (or recount) text
   As we saw in Chapter 7, descriptive text can be categorised into three structures: list, web, and compare-contrast. Other structures include hierarchy.

   a. List structure
      A text with a *list structure* lays out information like a shopping list, such as a list of products made in a country or a list of materials found in a rubbish dump. There is no clear link between the items of information.

   b. Web structure
      The information in factual text may be about one thing that can be put into categories. For example, the information in a text about Tasmanian tigers might be in clusters of information such as habitat, diet, descriptive features and enemies, which forms a *web structure*. An example of a web structure for writing is given in Figure 8.5, where a Year 6 student is writing about dogs. It is a web because it is about just one thing. Prior to writing, the class had read an article about dogs and brainstormed some ideas.

Figure 8.5: Dogs – students read an article about dogs and brainstormed some ideas for an article that explains about dogs to someone who does not know much about dogs

> Opens with a question – hooks the reader

> Features of dogs – e.g., size, kinds

> Friendly close to the article/ essay

Do you know much about dogs? If not then then you need my help. A dog is part of the canidae family. They love to play and go for runs, they can be big or small, loud or quiet. They are known as mans best friend. What girls love dogs too. They are a mamal. A mammal is a type of animal. The dog does not lay eggs the babbies grow in their tummy. The smalest dog is a Chihwahwas the biggest is the big dane. Smaller dogs live longer than big dogs. This I hope this has helped you know more about dogs.

In assessing the above piece of writing about "dogs", the first thing to note is that it lacks a title, but it has a good introduction that gets your attention and a good closing that reaches out to the reader. The middle section explains about a dog is part of the canidae family, games that dogs play, that they are mammals, as well as information on the size of dogs and their life span. In terms of conventions, it lacks paragraphing and there are some spelling mistakes. It would have been nice to use some categories like "features of dogs" and "types of dogs" but overall it is a good summary.

c. Compare-contrast structure

In a *compare–contrast structure* the information is about more than one thing, and there are direct comparisons and contrasts that can be made (e.g., the similarities and differences between Auckland and Melbourne, such as location, population, manufacturing industries, weather, and so on). Or, the text might compare two different kinds of bird by colour, size, diet and habitat, or two different kinds of car by engine size, shape, comfort, safety and reliability.

d. Hierarchy structure

In a *hierarchy structure* the information is presented by moving from the more general category to subcategories. For example, the top of the hierarchy could be animals, the next level down is kinds of animals (birds, insects, etc.), and the next level down could be kinds of birds (sparrows, seagulls, pigeons, hawks, etc.).

The next level down could then be information about each bird (such as features, habitat, food, enemies). This information (about habitat etc.) would then create a matrix within the hierarchical structure. Many articles are not just one structure but can have more than one structure within them.

Figure 8.6. A hierarchy structure for "Animals"

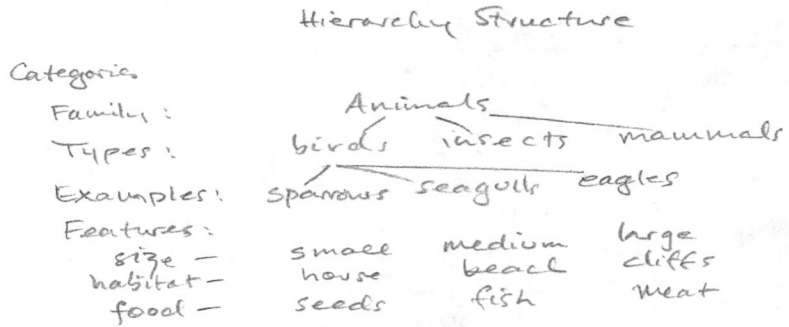

5. Sequential text
   There are three structures within sequential text:
   - linear
   - cause–effect
   - problem–solution.

In text with a *linear structure*, one thing happens after the other (e.g., the steps in making a cake, milking a cow, starting a computer). In a cause–effect structure one event causes another to happen (e.g., an earthquake causes the ground to move, which then causes buildings to collapse, and people to get hurt, and so on).
Finally, in a problem–solution structure a problem is presented and solutions are offered. For example, a historic building may be located on valuable inner-city land where a developer wants to build a supermarket. Possible solutions are to find another location for the supermarket, or move the historic building to another place, or destroy the building.

Figure 8.7 A problem–solution structure for the problem of how to keep an historic building but still have a supermarket on valuable land

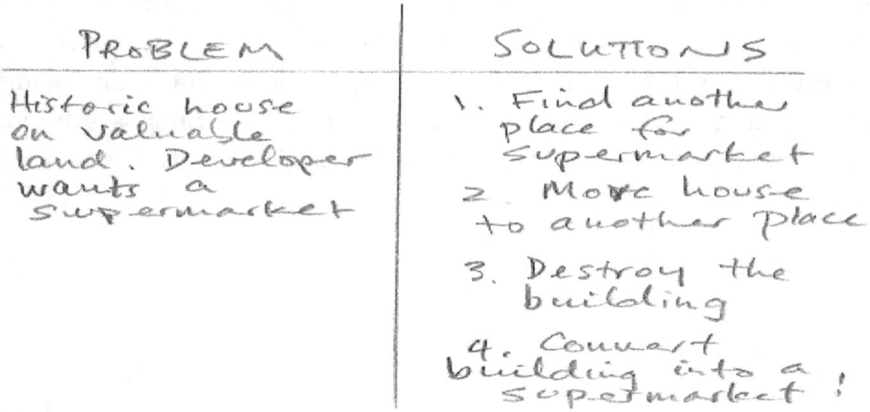

PROBLEM	SOLUTIONS
Historic house on valuable land. Developer wants a supermarket	1. Find another place for supermarket 2. Move house to another place 3. Destroy the building 4. Convert building into a supermarket!

6. Persuasive text
    Normally persuasive text gives information for and against an idea, but sometimes the information may be one-sided, as in advertising, where the information about a product is usually positive. Writers who can persuade are able to consider the audience and predict how well the audience will receive their ideas. These are the skills of persuasion. The skills involve being:
    - aware that the audience might disagree
    - aware that opinions will differ.

A persuasive speech or essay needs to be well thought out. Suggest to your students that they state their position right up front, present their arguments in the middle, and at the end of the essay try to get the audience onside with a personal plea or a prediction, or simply sum up what they have said.

For example, if they are writing a persuasive piece on the topic of why all children should play sport, they can brainstorm a number of reasons related to fitness, social interaction, and so on. They can mention downsides like injuries, but counter that with sports where there are not so many injuries.

Novice writers are less likely to seek compromise: 'The rainforests must be saved at all costs!' As students make progress in their skills there is more use of compromise in their writing. A more effective piece of persuasive writing uses negotiation markers and counter-arguments, and shows more of a sense of obligation (e.g., 'We should save the rain forests because it is a good thing to do'). It will also show more indicators of uncertainty, using words such as *maybe* and *surely*.

Summary

Students with dyslexia often have good ideas for writing, but often it takes ages to get their ideas down on paper because they struggle with the mechanics of writing (i.e., spelling). This is why we need to encourage accurate and fluent spelling. This does not mean that spelling is sufficient. The simple view of writing says that ideas are important as well, and we have suggested some strategies to make this happen.

CHAPTER 9

The importance of fluency and how to teach it effectively

What is reading fluency?

Fluency is critical for reading with understanding. Fluent reading can be reading aloud or silent reading. It refers to our ability to process text accurately and quickly at a rate that enables comprehension as well. It is not helter-skelter reading where you are sprinting along the lines of text. It is not skim reading or scanning just the subheadings or topic sentences of text. It is reading every word in the text about as fast as you usually listen, at a conversational rate, and with understanding.

A definition of reading fluency is the ability to read with speed and accuracy at a conversational rate. If the reading task involves reading aloud, fluency also includes being able to read with expression in an engaging way not in a dull monotone (National Institute of Child Health and Human Development, 2000a; Therrien, 2004).

We are not always able to read fluently. If the material is difficult, even if we are fluent readers we have to change down through the gears and our reading is slower. For normal reading, though, we tend to read at a fixed rate, for example, Carver (1992) wrote that a grade 6 female pupil (11–12 years old) would read her history textbook at fairly steady rate of 177 words a minute. Fluent reading is reading at a reasonable speed that allows comprehension.

This seems a simple explanation of fluency, but many researchers say it is deceptive because reading fluency involves a range of skills (Hudson, Pullen, Lane, & Torgesen, 2009). When you are reading fluently, you are decoding and comprehending. This is not always the case when you are reading. You can read the words in a text accurately but may not understand what you are reading. This could be because the meaning is difficult or it might be because the task only requires you to decode, so your mind is not on comprehension but on making a nice presentation. We probably all remember as children reading aloud to the teacher with expression but not really thinking about the meaning while doing it. Instead, we were focusing on presenting well. This is not fluent reading. Fluency involves reading with understanding.

An important aspect of fluency is automaticity, this is the ability to read words effortlessly, using very little mental energy for decoding words, so as to be able to concentrate fully on the meaning of the text (Eldridge, 2005). Students who have reading difficulties perform much worse in fluency than students who are not classified as having reading difficulties, mainly because of their difficulties with decoding (Wanzek, Al Otaiba, & Petscher, 2014).

The reading speeds of children and adults

Reading fluency doesn't happen overnight. It takes a long time for students to reach a reading speed similar to that of an adult. Adults read at 200 words per minute or more; school students do not get near to this level until they are in high school (Carver, 1990). This is not a criticism of our teaching of reading but an acknowledgement that it is not easy to become fluent in reading. The positive is that students gradually improve in reading fluency over time. Hughes and Wilkins (2000) reported a study of 120 pupils who read passages aloud and approximate oral reading speeds were:

- 5 years: 60–70 words per minute
- 6 years: 90 words per minute
- 7 years: 100 words per minute
- 8 years: 110 words per minute
- 9 years: 120 words per minute.

Note: Hughes and Wilkins (2000) found variation in reading speed for 5- to 7-year-olds depending on the size of the print. Younger children read faster with slightly larger print.

Research on fluency

Research on fluency has a long history, going back four decades at least. There are two views about how fluency happens. One is that fluency reflects *decoding skills*: fast and accurate decoding enables easy word processing (which helps the flow of thought and increases comprehension) whereas slow decoding causes a bottleneck in processing (which slows the flow of thought and interrupts comprehension) (LaBerge & Samuels, 1974; Samuels, 1979).

Another view is that reading without fluency is not caused by poor decoding alone, but also reflects difficulty in using prosodic cues, such as punctuation. Lack of prosody can also interfere with comprehension. The ability to use prosodic cues is shown when the reader pauses at the right places in the text, raises their voice for exclamation marks or for bolded print, stresses the right words in clauses, and so on. Does this mean that the ability to use prosodic cues increases fluency? Eldridge (2005) thought it might be a result of fluency rather than a cause. If you are fluent you are usually good at using prosodic cues in the text to read with expression.

Clay and Imlach (1971) in New Zealand found that good readers showed much more use of prosodic cues when reading aloud than did poor readers. In their study they assessed 103 7-year-old children. They chose four stories for the children to read, each one harder than the one before. Children read for 10 minutes, or until they finished all the stories. Above average readers read an average of 907 words, with an error rate of less than 1 percent. In contrast, below-average readers read 212 words with an error rate of 34 percent. The above-average readers read at 100 words per minute, while the below-average readers read at 14 words per minute. The above-average readers made much more use of prosodic cues: they paused more at the ends of sentences, after commas, and so on. It seemed that the fluency of the above-average readers was due to their use of prosodic cues, but it could be that their much better fluency caused their better use of prosodic cues. When you think about it, the above-average readers were faster at reading and this is a sign of fluency whereas the below-average readers were much slower, indicating the material they were reading was way too hard for them. They were not able to be fluent with such hard material so they could not read with expression either. It is that chicken-egg problem.

This is the puzzle with the prosody view of fluency: it is hard to know if the pupil is fluent because they attend to prosodic cues, or if the pupil is better able to attend to prosodic cues because they are fluent. The teacher would need to sort out whether the lack of attention to prosody is because the material is too difficult. Giving them easier material to read might produce a much different reader who is fluent and has prosody as well.

Teaching fluency through reading connected text

Repeated reading

One approach that does have a large research base is the strategy of repeated reading. Not every repeated reading strategy works, though. Therrien (2004) reviewed the literature on different repeated reading approaches and found that some have little research support. These were the neurological impress method, where the student and teacher read aloud together; assisted reading, or reading while listening, where the student reads along with an audiotape instead of a person; and paired reading, where the student reads along with a better reader (it could be a classmate or an adult) until they are ready to read alone.

After reviewing a number of repeated reading studies, Therrien (2004) found that often they did not have a control group, which violates one of the golden rules for scientific studies, because it means the results could be due to other factors, such as the novelty effect of being in a research study. Even so, from the evidence available, Therrien concluded that if teachers want to use repeated reading to increase fluency and comprehension, the features of the strategy should be to:

- read aloud to an adult (not a peer)
- give corrective feedback on miscues
- use a performance criterion (e.g., the pupil has to keep reading the text until he/she is able to read at 100 words per minute)
- read the text more than twice.

The repeated reading approach involves reading the same text several times until the student achieves fluency. Reviews of research on this strategy have been positive, with small to moderate effect sizes* of .55 for accuracy, .44 for fluency and .35 for reading comprehension (National Institute of Child Health and Human Development, 2000a), though the NRP report cautioned about small sample sizes in the studies they reviewed. A moderate or large effect size means it is definitely worth trying in the classroom.

Therrien (2004) reported a meta-analysis based on 18 studies of repeated reading. The aim of the analysis was to find out the effects of repeated reading. The meta-analytic review showed that the repeated reading strategy worked well for specific texts that were repeatedly read, with large effect sizes for fluency (.83) moderate for comprehension (.67), but for texts the student had not read before the effect sizes were moderate for fluency (.50) and small for comprehension (.25).

The effect sizes for reading specific texts they had read before in repeated reading (i.e. 'non-transfer' texts) varied according to the features of the repeated reading. For these

---

* Effect size is a statistical term that describes the size of the relationship between two variables. Effect sizes can be small (.2 to .4), medium (.5 to .7) or large (.8 or more).

texts it did not seem to matter if the student was cued to read for speed, or comprehension, or both; the effect sizes were similar. If the student received feedback on their miscues while reading, this reduced their fluency. If the student read the text multiple times (up to four times), effect sizes were large for fluency and moderate for comprehension.

The effect sizes for reading new texts students had not read before (i.e. 'transfer' texts) varied depending on the features of the repeated reading strategy. The effect sizes were moderate to large if the repeated reading was to an adult (fluency 1.37, comprehension .71) whereas if students read to a peer the effect sizes were small (fluency .36, comprehension .22).

Modelling by peers, where the tutor read the text before the tutee read it, seemed to interfere with comprehension for the tutee. Receiving corrective feedback on miscues while reading had small effects on fluency and comprehension if given by the peer tutor, but large effects if given by adults (there were no data for comprehension when adults were tutors). There was a large effect for fluency if the student had to reach a criterion, such as a certain number of words read per minute. There was also a moderate effect for fluency and comprehension if the student read the text two or three times.

So, does repeated reading really work for pupils with reading difficulties? A cautionary note comes from a review of 11 repeated reading studies focusing on students with reading difficulties (Chard, Ketterlin-Geller, Baker, Doabler, & Apichatabutra, 2009). There were six single-subject studies (a sample of one or a few pupils but with repeated measurements of their progress) and five experimental studies (where the sample size is usually larger and there is a treatment group and often a control group). The studies were looked at in terms of criteria for being evidence-based. The researchers concluded, though, that the studies could not be called evidence-based because there were too many research problems, such as the possibility of teacher effects (different teachers in one group and the other), lack of treatment fidelity checks (not checking to see if the treatment was done correctly), no replication (only one study), lack of control groups (a comparison group that is matched or very similar in ability), and not using a general measure of reading fluency (a measure that used different texts to the ones used in the study). These problems suggest that we have to be cautious about accepting too easily the research on repeated readings.

Sustained silent reading in the classroom

One way to increase fluency might be to have reading practice in the classroom, as in sustained silent reading (SSR), where students spend time each day reading silently on their own. It seems logical that reading practice (or reading 'mileage') will improve reading achievement, but the report of the National Reading Panel in the United States (National Institute of Child Health and Human Development. 2000a) concluded:

Based on the existing evidence, the NRP can only indicate that while encouraging students to read might be beneficial, research has not yet demonstrated this in a clear and convincing manner. (p. 3)

A problem with SSR is that there is no way to verify that students are reading rather than simply looking at the pictures or day-dreaming; so much of the time students doing SSR might be looking at the page but their attention is elsewhere (Garan & DeVoogd, 2008; Widdowson, Moore, & Dixon, 1998). This is particularly true for struggling readers, who may not want to read even though there is free time for them to do it. The NRP (2000a) report did not find enough evidence to come to firm conclusions about the benefits of SSR for fluency.

Good readers read much more than poor readers, and it seems logical that if poor readers also did more reading they would improve in reading, but it may be that the reason good readers read more is not that they read more but that they are skilled at reading words, so reading is not a chore for them. Asking poor readers to do SSR may frustrate them and not help them if they cannot read very well.

Would SSR be easier if the material was at their reading level? Reutzel, Petscher and Spichtig (2008) looked at this idea in a study with 80 third-grade struggling readers, where the experimental group received computerised reading practice at their reading level. They called it guided oral reading practice, in that the computer program had a variety of stories and tasks that could keep the students' interest. The results were mixed: the computer practice group was better on an informal reading test than a control group, but there was no difference between them and the control group on a standardised reading test. In other words, there was no clear advantage for guided oral reading.

Researchers have found that students who need the most practice in reading do the least amount of reading (Allington, 1977, 2013; Allington & Gabriel, 2012), so we need to find ways to increase reading practice. Reading material where the pupil makes very few errors may be important for fluency. Allington (2013) suggests a level of 98 percent accuracy, which is material that is very easy to read. A number of studies suggest that reading at the right level improves student behaviour and motivation (Allington, 2013).

Reading aloud to someone at independent or instructional level does help to improve oral reading fluency and reading comprehension (O'Connor, Swanson, & Geraghty, 2010). Reading aloud to another person avoids the big problem of SSR, in that when you are reading to someone you *have* to engage with the text and your mind is not allowed to wander, as can happen in SSR. There is some evidence to support reading aloud to another person. Forty-five minutes of reading practice a week in three 15-minute sessions for 14 weeks, with someone listening to you read and giving feedback about errors was shown to improve fluency and reading comprehension (O'Connor, White, & Swanson, 2007). Other researchers have obtained similar results (Shany & Biemiller, 1995).

Big Book reading

Big Books are usually used with Year 1–2 students but we have seen them used with Year 6 classes as well. The text is BIG with enlarged print so all the class can see the words (for more detail, see Tse & Nicholson, 2014). Big Book reading includes repeated reading and a focus on fluency, where the teacher provides instruction in how to use prosodic cues such as punctuation, helps with the decoding of words, and encourages comprehension. The fluency aspect of Big Book reading is that the teacher reads the same book, usually on four different days of the week, which is a key feature of the repeated reading approach. Eldridge, Reutzel and Hollingsworth (1996) compared Big Book reading with round-robin reading. In their study, round-robin reading was, where the teacher took children in small groups and had each of them read aloud to her. Another form of round robin reading they studied was reading aloud to a buddy. They found that Big Book reading produced bigger gains in accuracy, comprehension and fluency.

Big Book reading effectiveness probably also depends on the extent to which children engage with the text. Some studies indicate that younger pupils do not look much at the text unless it is easier for them to decode. Instead, they look at the illustrations. Researchers studying the eye movements of children from kindergarten through fourth grade (Evans & Saint-Aubin, 2013; Roy-Charland, Saint-Aubin, & Evans, 2007) found that kindergarten children from high socioeconomic circumstances spent less than 10 percent of the time looking at the text—they looked at the illustrations. They found that children did learn new vocabulary (the better their own vocabulary, the more words they learned), but shared book reading did not help their reading. In grade 1, children spent more time looking at the text as long as the text was easy for them.

In grades 2–4 children spent about half the time looking at the text while the teacher was reading (from 45 to 65 percent), so they were partially reading along with the print as the teacher or parent read the book to them. This is probably because at that stage they had some decoding skill and could process the print. The researchers concluded that older children can benefit from shared book reading in terms of fluency if the text is easy for them to read. If the text is too hard, they don't look at the print and are unlikely to benefit.

Fluency and Big Book reading

Big Book reading may be a way to increase fluency. The Big Book is usually read several times in class so it offers repeated reading practice. Tse and Nicholson (2014) reported a study in which 6-year-old average and below-average readers from disadvantaged backgrounds engaged in Big Book reading that was enhanced with phonics and phonemic awareness. The study found that this combined approach was just as effective as Big Book reading on its own for passage reading accuracy and just as effective as phonics on its own for basic decoding skills but it was more effective than either Big Book reading or phonics on their own for other literacy measures including reading comprehension, word reading, phonemic awareness, and spelling. Although the study did not measure fluency, the combined approach may be a useful way to help students build fluency because it improves word reading skills and this may make it easier to build accurate and fast reading. Some examples of combined lessons from the study are included in Appendix 8.

Teaching fluency by developing sub-skills

Eldridge (2005) assessed the reading skills of 233 first- to third-grade students and found positive correlations between phonics skills and word recognition ($r = .43$ to $.55$) and between word recognition and fluency ($r = .75$ to $.84$). This indicated that fluency is a result of good skills in word recognition (Hudson et al., 2009). The easier it is to read words, the faster you will read. Poor readers usually lack good word recognition skills, and it makes sense that we should focus on building these before, or at least at the same time as, trying to improve fluency (Pikulski & Chard, 2005).

Teaching basic decoding skills

Iversen and Tunmer (1993) used the 'make and break' technique successfully to do this with 6-year-olds who were struggling. This technique is now part of Reading Recovery teaching. In this technique, the teacher uses magnetic letters (a good set of these is provided in *Teaching Phonics Effectively*, published by Smart Kids). Alternatively, the teacher can use a whiteboard and pen with the pupil. It goes like this (as explained in Iversen & Tunmer, 1993). The teacher makes the word *and* with magnetic letters, then asks the pupil, 'What does this say?' The teacher jumbles up the letters and the pupil has to reconstruct the word *and*. The teacher shows them if the pupil does not know. Then the teacher asks, 'What word did you just make?' This is repeated until the pupil can do it. The teacher puts an *s* in front of *and*, then shows how the word works by running her finger from *s* through to the end of the word. He or she then takes away the *s* and explains that this now says *and* and asks the pupil to make *sand*. The teacher asks, 'What word have you made?' This is repeated until the pupil gets the idea.

The teacher then asks the pupil to make *and*, *hand*, *sand* and *band*. This is repeated with other words until the pupil gets the idea that changing letters will change the word. The teacher at a later stage asks the pupil to change other aspects of the word, such as changing *hat* to *that* to *pat* to *sat* to *sit* to *hit* to *hut*, and so on. The teacher not only does this for reading but also for spelling, asking the pupil to spell *and*, *sand*, and so on.

Teaching pupils to read words faster

There is research to support practice in reading high frequency words as a way to help fluency. Ring, Barefoot, Avrit, Brown and Black (2013) taught students in grades 1–5 to practise both word reading and text reading. They found that both kinds of practice had similar positive effects on fluency but that the word reading practice had better effects on reading accuracy than did text reading practice. Watts and Gardner (2013) found a significant benefit from teaching a set of 113 high-frequency words for 5 minutes a day for 5 weeks to a small group of eight Year 1 pupils, some of whom were struggling with reading; all pupils improved in speed and accuracy.

Reading of text

Reading books independently is a great way to build fluency through reading practice. It is important that the reading material is easy enough to read with high levels of accuracy (Allington, 2013). A suggestion is to try the high interest books recommended in Nicholson & Dymock (2010). This list is graded from primary to secondary school level so the pupil can select books that are not too hard for them. There are also apps on the market that have reading materials graded in levels of difficulty so students can choose to read texts that are not too difficult, for example, see the list below:

1. Spin Out stories – for secondary school students (not graded but high interest)
2. Fitzroy readers – graded – books 1–40 – phonics readers
3. Oxford owls – graded – 250 free books (you have to register first)
4. Sunshine Classics – graded
5. Read Me Stories – graded

Summary

To sum up, repeated reading of text or simply extensive reading of text will build reading fluency but it is important for students to have good decoding skills to get the full benefit of reading practice. The benefits are more likely if students are reading text at the right difficulty level—preferably very easy to read—so they can put into practice the word skills they have learned by reading words in context. Big Book reading and reading of lots of material at the right difficulty level will provide that practice. Book Book reading at school provides repeated reading of the text in that the same text is normally read three or four times during the school week by the teacher to and with the class.

It is better if the student is reading to someone, as in oral reading to the teacher or their parents, rather than listening to someone else read to them, because it engages them in reading and they focus on the words in the text and not so much the illustrations. Reading aloud also provides essential reading practice.

CHAPTER 10

Making the classroom a dyslexia-friendly place

Introduction

A dyslexia-friendly classroom is about changing how the curriculum is presented so that it is friendlier. Such a classroom is one where any student with reading difficulties is likely to feel welcome and supported. How do you do this? In the Introduction we reported on a survey of the British general public (Whitehead, 2007) showing that three-quarters understood little or nothing about dyslexia, one in five thought dyslexics just need to work harder, and half thought dyslexia is just getting words and letters back to front.

We also reported in Chapter 3 on two surveys of schools in the Waikato and Auckland area showing that 20 of 68 respondents (29 percent) felt equipped to deal with dyslexia. These results suggest that many teachers are seeking ideas on how to help students with dyslexia. This chapter is about how to make changes in the classroom. Hopefully these ideas will be taken up in the wider workplace as well.

What makes for a dyslexia-friendly classroom?

Coffield, Riddick, Barmby and O'Neill (2008) surveyed 18 primary schools in the UK on the dyslexia friendliness of their classroom and teachers. The questionnaire covered classroom practices, whether they enjoyed school, and how they felt in class. A sample of 104 Year 2 to 6 students completed the survey; 43 students had dyslexia, 8 students had special educational needs, and 53 students did not have dyslexia or special needs. The survey data from the 43 students with dyslexia were analysed separately.

Students with dyslexia identified things they hated, which were: bullying, teachers shouting, and teachers getting mad or bossy. The dyslexic students (43 of the 104 students surveyed) also felt that teachers provided support in four ways (Coffield et al., 2008):

- reading important text to the class (65 percent of students with dyslexia)
- providing support material such as special dictionaries and word mats (57 percent of students with dyslexia)
- showing willingness to repeat instructions (53 percent of students with dyslexia)
- developing easy-to-follow worksheets where important information is highlighted (45 percent of students with dyslexia).

Students without dyslexia also identified these strategies, in similar proportions, as ways teachers provided support. Coffield et al. (2008) also found that 35 percent of students in the study lacked the confidence to read out loud in class, 54 percent received "lots of red marks" (p. 359) in their exercise books, and 21 percent reported that they were not given enough time to write their homework. Students with dyslexia believed that they were more likely to "get in trouble" if they did not bring the right equipment to their lessons.

These things can be easily remedied in the classroom. Careful consideration needs to be given when asking students to read aloud. Students with dyslexia, or students with reading difficulties, report that reading aloud is an unpleasant experience (refer to 'Ryan's story' in this book's companion video *Talking about Dyslexia*: see www.nzcer.org.nz/nzcerpress/new-zealand-dyslexia-handbook). Why would a teacher ask a child with dyslexia to read in front of their peers? Teachers should avoid giving red marks for all the errors the student makes. Instead, teachers should identify a few things the student needs to focus on. Giving an extension of time for classwork, or accepting one paragraph instead of two, or not punishing a child for not finishing their work is a step in the direction of a dyslexia-friendly classroom (refer to William's comments on not having enough time to complete work in 'William's story').

Following is a description of five things to avoid when you have a dyslexic student.

> **Five things to avoid when you have a student with dyslexia**
>
> 1. Don't ask poor readers to read out loud in front of the class, or in small groups. One adult with dyslexia said, "I got slung out of school eventually. I was told to read just once too often, then someone laughed when I couldn't pronounce things right and I lost it. Thumped him, threw stuff, threatened the teacher. It was sort of downhill from there" (Mortimore & Dupree, 2008, p. 16).
>
> 2. Don't ask a classmate to correct their spelling test (i.e., don't swap tests and mark), because it reveals to another student their spelling ability. Poor spellers do not like it when their peers discover they have spelling difficulties.
>
> 3. Don't ask poor spellers to write on the whiteboard. It is like round robin reading or reading aloud to the class: it simply shows their peer group that they have spelling difficulties.
>
> 4. Don't ask poor readers to read an article or story in too short a time frame. It is like asking a good reader to read a novel in an hour. Students with dyslexia need more time. Give the student the article or story the day before and explain to them that the class or group will be discussing it the following day. One of our students found it very frustrating when the teacher gave the class or group a limited amount of time to read an article or chapter in content area reading. By the time he had read the first page most of the class had finished the article/chapter and were ready to discuss the content. The student was then cut out of the conversation.
>
> 5. Don't give long lists of spelling words to learn. An adult with dyslexia reflecting on her school days said that due to the stress associated with learning the lists of words, "In the end I stopped going on spelling test days" (Mortimore & Dupree, 2008, p. 16). Another adult with dyslexia commented on the teacher's written comments: one was "check your spelling". The response, "I only wish I could" (Mortimore & Dupree, 2008, p. 17).

What other things can primary teachers do to make their class dyslexia friendly?

Seating arrangements

One of the authors visited Benchmark School in Media, Pennsylvania, which is a school for children experiencing reading difficulties, many with dyslexia. A teacher of 8-year-old children was asked about her classroom seating arrangement. The teacher replied that two of the students with the greatest learning need sat in the back row in the inner aisle seats. The students were placed there so the teacher could kneel down to help both students yet still have an eye on the rest of the class (see the white seats in Figure 10.1 below). The student in the red seat was positioned here so that he could slip out of the classroom to work with a specialist teacher. His placement meant he did not have to disturb other students, nor was he noticed by fellow students as he left the room, as the door was close to his desk. When organising seating arrangements the Benchmark School teacher considered both classroom management (e.g., being able to see all children when helping students that required the most support) and minimising the disruption of learning due to students moving in and out of the classroom.

Figure 10.1: One suggested classroom seating arrangement

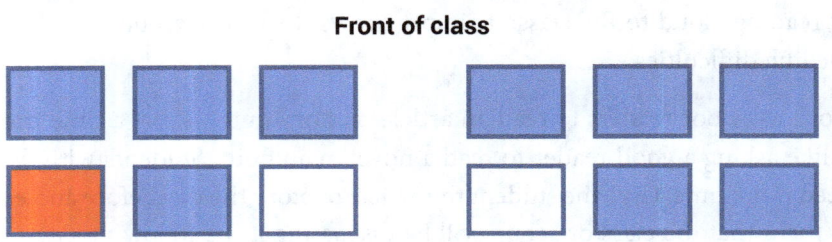

In contrast to the arrangements at Benchmark School, the British Dyslexia Association (BDA) (2006) recommends a seating arrangement where pupils with dyslexia sit at the front of the class, next to a buddy or peer mentor, and away from distractions, so the teacher can monitor how they cope with class work. Sitting near the classroom door, for example, would be a distraction, as would sitting near the classroom sink, class library, and class computers. In our interview with William (see "the Dyslexia Friendly Classroom" in this book's companion video), he told us he preferred to sit near the front of the class. Thus, unless there is an issue with a dyslexic pupil often having to leave the classroom for extra help, and therefore needing to be near the classroom door, it is better that pupils with dyslexia sit near the front of the room but away from all distractions.

Asking for help

Asking a classmate for help is a strategy that some of the primary and secondary students we have taught in the Hamilton Children's Reading Centre use to help cope with academic demands. Help could be in the form of reading the question or clarifying instructions. One of our secondary students struck up a deal with a classmate. The deal was that his friend would read the question and the student with dyslexia would tell him the answer. A primary student we taught made the decision to ask a number of students to assist him so as not to burden one student. He also commented that he did not like "bugging" or "interrupting" other students, and so there were times when he did not ask for help.

Copying from the whiteboard

According to the BDA (2006), copying from a whiteboard is challenging for the student with dyslexia due to their difficulties with spelling and the time it takes them to write. Students may copy one or two letters at a time. Each time they return to what may appear as a 'crowded' whiteboard they can easily lose their place. Teachers should consider using the whiteboard for key points rather than for a lot of writing.

Other dyslexia-friendly classroom ideas

Keep expectations appropriate for the student. Dyslexia robs you of time (Shaywitz, 2003), so if the class is given 15–20 minutes to write a descriptive paragraph about the class rabbit, it could be that the student with dyslexia will only write a couple of sentences. Do not expect the same quantity of work as their non-dyslexic counterparts provide.

Set homework that is achievable for students with dyslexia, knowing that they will take longer to complete it. Hattie (2009, p. 234) reports that while homework is a "hotly contested area", the "overall effects [of homework] are positive". Hattie reported that "task-oriented homework had higher effects than deep learning and problem solving homework" (p. 235). Hattie also found that effects were higher for maths homework than for science or social studies, and higher when "the material was not complex or if it was novel", and that the effects of homework were greater for more able students and for older students and secondary students compared to primary students. Hattie (2009) does, however, caution that

> for too many students, homework reinforces that they cannot learn by themselves, and that they cannot do the schoolwork. For these students, homework can undermine motivation, internalise incorrect routines and strategies, and reinforce less effective study habits, especially for elementary students. (p. 235)

Setting homework often seems to be setting poor readers up for failure. Homework for the student with dyslexia is not going to end well unless they can buddy up with a good reader who can help them, go through the assignment with them, and work together to get a solution to the problem set.

The need for trust

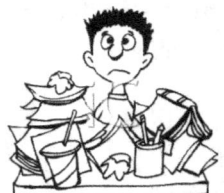

In one intermediate classroom we visited, the teacher did her best to ensure the needs of all children were met (refer to the 'Dyslexia friendly classroom' in this book's companion video *Talking about Dyslexia* (see www.nzcer.org.nz/nzcerpress/new-zealand-dyslexia-handbook)). A key goal for the first few weeks of term 1 was to build an environment of trust so that all students felt safe. For the students with dyslexia she:

- placed them close to the whiteboard.
- considered the size, shape and spacing of print when writing on the whiteboard
- ensured the font size on hand-outs was large and easy to read and not crammed with information or assignment details
- included a lot of collaboration, where the students worked together in groups
- arranged a reader-writer for tests (the student would often complete the test twice; particularly standardised tests like e-asTTle) first independently, and the second time with a reader-writer
- placed students with dyslexia in reading groups according to language comprehension ability, rather than decoding ability, because she knew they were able to understand class content if it was in a discussion format.

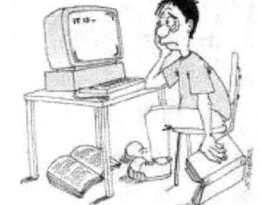

The Year 8 teacher found that the student with dyslexia she taught preferred a routine (e.g., maths after interval), but knowing that routines at secondary school often change and students need to be able to adapt to change when they arrive in high school, occasionally during the second half of the year she altered the classroom routine (e.g., maths before interval). She explained that the change in routine was to prepare them for high school. This enabled students to experience change in a safe environment.

The secondary school classroom

Stories of students with dyslexia

Jade

Jade's poor decoding and encoding skills were not addressed during his 11 years of compulsory schooling. At the age of 16, disillusioned and more or less told he was no longer welcome at school, he left with no formal qualification. Jade's language comprehension was good, he could understand text material if it was read to him, and he had good ideas to write about, but he was poor at reading and recording his thoughts. In Jade's case his difficulties meant that he did not get a school qualification even though he had good language skills.

Ariana

Ariana had good language skills and good maths skills but was poor at spelling and decoding words, fitting the profile of dyslexia. She left high school with NCEA Levels 1, 2 and 3. She has since enrolled in a course at a private training establishment (PTE). She was referred to the literacy tutor at the PTE because she had decoding and spelling difficulties. Her tutor commented, "She can't write a sentence without mistakes" (Personal communication, 22 March 2013). Ariana's profile is not too different to Jade's, although unlike Jade, Ariana left school with a qualification.

Forward planning and awareness of dyslexia: two dyslexia-friendly principles for the secondary school classroom

Gavin Reid (2010) suggests that if secondary schools are going to meet the needs of students with dyslexia, *all staff* need to consider the needs of this group of students. It is not enough for one, two or some teachers/staff to meet the needs of students with dyslexia. The school, as a whole, needs to be supportive. Reid (2010) argues that there are two key dyslexia-friendly principles that are applicable to all curriculum areas: "forward planning" and an "awareness of dyslexia" (Reid, 2010, p. 99)

PRINCIPLE 1: Forward planning

In this context, forward planning is planning undertaken by the teacher prior to teaching so that the needs of students with dyslexia are catered for. Dyslexic students experience difficulty with reading and writing, ranging from mild to severe. Some, as the result of specialist tuition, are able to read with accuracy but not fluency. That is, some dyslexic students are able to decode, but they do so with much effort. Due to dyslexia some students read with accuracy 1 to 2 years below their age level, and others who are affected more severely decode 4 or more years below their chronological age.

What are the practical steps teachers should consider to create a dyslexia-friendly secondary classroom? Students with dyslexia have good vocabularies and good listening skills. If the text is read to them, or if they are able to follow along in read-along style, comprehension is good.

Forward planning suggestions

(a) For the student with poor decoding skills (both accuracy and fluency)
- Distribute a copy of the text in advance (at least a day).
- Provide an audio recording of the text (e.g., a software program that enables the student to also listen to the text).
- Read the text aloud.
- When writing on the whiteboard, read the text as you write.

- Background knowledge plays an important role in reading comprehension. Build background knowledge prior to reading, so that when the student with dyslexia encounters a difficult word, they can use context to decode. Context is not a particularly reliable decoding strategy, but at times it is helpful (Nicholson & Dymock, 2010).
- Break the task into smaller chunks (e.g., part of a chapter or article).
- Source text with visual aids (e.g., diagrams, charts, illustrations).

(b) For the student who decodes with accuracy but lacks fluency

This student is able to read age-appropriate texts but requires more time to process.
- Distribute a copy of the text in advance (at least a day).
- Break the task into smaller chunks (e.g., part of a chapter or article).
- Source text with visual aids (e.g., diagrams, charts, illustrations).

(c) For a student with good decoding skills (age appropriate or higher) but poor spelling

This student is able to read and process written text at a similar speed as his classmates but his spelling and writing fluency are poor.
- Make available speech-to-text software.
- Focus on quality rather than quantity (e.g., explain to the student that one rather than two pages is required).
- Source a suitable dictionary (appropriate for age *and* spelling level).
- Use a computer rather than hand writing. Students can then use a spell checker. Note that spell checking is not a guarantee that the correct words are used (e.g., sea or see; break or brake).

Reid (2010, p. 107) suggests that forward planning for high school students with dyslexia should include (abridged):
- knowing the readability level of the text and the reading level of the student—is the text close to the reading level of the student or is the gap wide (e.g., more than 12–18 months)?
- avoiding text that is 'dense'—source text with diagrams, charts, illustrations
- providing notes, PowerPoint, headings, so that students do not have to take a lot of notes, allowing the student to concentrate on what is being said
- providing specialised vocabulary lists (particularly in the content area)
- arranging software for the student (text-to-speech, speech-to-text) http://www.naturalreaders.com/
- sourcing material that is audio-recorded:
  - http://ebook-reader-review.toptenreviews.com/
  - plus thousands of books are available as audio-books (English).

Reid argues that there are a number of key issues for the student (2010, p. 107):
- ensuring the content is accessible
- presenting the content in a dyslexia-friendly way
- including a range of assessment types
- providing professional development for staff.

PRINCIPLE 2: Awareness of dyslexia

Understanding the characteristics and nature of dyslexia is the first step to being able to cater for students with dyslexia. The next step is knowing how to screen for dyslexia. Although the classroom teacher might not be able to formally assess a student for dyslexia, they can screen for dyslexia. Having an awareness of the student's strengths and areas needing support will enable the teacher to plan an appropriate programme.

Mortimore and Dupree (2008) have established a set of *ground rules* for dyslexia-friendly classrooms. Their ground rules are aimed at encouraging students' strengths, which they argue (p. 41) means:
- not exposing the students' weaknesses
- providing opportunities for success, however small, followed by praise, although they caution against 'hollow praise'—students will see straight through this
- ensuring students are aware of the progress they are making
- encouraging all students to think and talk about the ways in which they learn, and then allowing them to use their preferences and strengths whenever possible
- encouraging students to explain their difficulties to the teacher, teacher's assistant or supportive peer/s so that teachers can co-operate to find the best ways to support students to develop independent strategies
- establishing a 'fairly steady' routine to create security and ensure that all students have taken in the instructions given
- being prepared to explain many times, in many ways, without publicising a student's failure to understand
- not expecting a student with dyslexia to be able to do two things at once (e.g., write and absorb instructions).

Never forget how embarrassing failure is. An important question researchers such as Riddick (2006) and Coffield et al. (2008) have asked is how a classroom is friendly enough to meet the needs of students with dyslexia. Coffield et al. claim that putting one or two strategies in place (e.g., reading instructions or less homework) is not adequate. They also remind us that the needs of students with dyslexia are not all the same. While some students liked being praised for their work, others did not like being singled out.

Appendix 9 is a survey Coffield et al. (2008) used to find out more about their students. You might like to use or adapt the survey to suit your needs. We think it will provide useful insights into the needs of your students.

Accommodation and modification

Wadlington, Jacob and Bailey (1996) argue that teachers should keep in mind 'accommodation' and 'modification' when considering their classroom environment and classroom programmes, as well as how the content is presented. 'Accommodation' refers to a change that enables the student to demonstrate what they have learned, such as more time to complete the test or a short break during an exam. It is something the teacher "does differently" (Barton, 2003, p. 10). Modification is where the task itself is modified. For example, the word limit may be reduced, or an oral rather than a written report presented.

The International Dyslexia Association (IDA) (2013) has produced a booklet for classroom teachers, *Dyslexia in the Classroom*. The booklet contains three sections: 'Accommodations involving materials' (pp. 7–8), 'Accommodations involving interactive instruction' (pp. 8–9) and 'Accommodations involving student performance' (pp. 9–10).

The IDA's recommendations for accommodations involving materials are to:
- clarify or simplify written instructions
- present a small amount of work
- block out extraneous stimuli
- highlight essential information
- provide additional practice activities
- provide a glossary in content areas
- develop reading guides
- use an audio-recording device
- use assistive technology.

Their recommendations relating to accommodations involving interactive instruction are to:
- use explicit teaching procedures
- repeat directions
- maintain daily routines
- provide a copy of lesson notes
- provide students with a graphic organiser
- use step-by-step instruction
- simultaneously combine verbal and visual information

- write key points or words on the whiteboard
- use mnemonic instruction
- emphasise daily review.

Finally, the recommendations for accommodations involving student performance are to:
- change the response mode (e.g., multi-choice rather than writing)
- provide an outline of the lesson
- encourage the use of graphic organisers
- place students close to the teacher
- encourage the use of calendars or assignment books
- use cues to denote important items
- design hierarchical worksheets (from easiest to hardest)
- allow the use of instructional aides (e.g., calculator, assistive technology)
- display work samples
- use peer-mediated learning
- use flexible work times
- provide additional practice
- use assignment substitutions or adjustments

Pull-out programmes: good or bad?

There are differing opinions on the effectiveness and overall benefits of pull-out programmes. Marston (1996) argues for a programme where students learn in their regular classroom but utilise "special instructional opportunities unavailable in general education" (p. 129). However, some students do not react well to the stigma associated with pull-out programmes. One of our students with dyslexia shared his experience of participating in such programmes. It was not unusual for him to be 'pulled out', with no prior warning. He would be working away at his desk, sometimes with other classmates, and a teacher would come to the classroom door and ask for him. He had to stand up, in front of his peers, and leave the room with the 'special' teacher. One day he refused to go, and an agreement was reached between the child and his teacher, and his later teachers, that he would not be pulled out of the classroom. He refused to be humiliated, yet again, in front of his peers.

Summary

There is a lot teachers can do to create dyslexia-friendly classrooms. We have suggested ideas that will make learning easier for students with dyslexia—in fact, easier for all students. The friendly classroom is where the teacher is flexible and takes into account the fact that struggling readers and writers are time-poor: they struggle to get their work done in time, or even at all, because they have difficulties reading and spelling. If there is a way to give them time, it *will* make a difference to them.

The classroom can be a place where they trust others and where they feel safe. Little accommodations the teacher makes do not have to be a lot of work for the teacher, but they can really help the student. Pull-out programmes can embarrass these pupils, especially as they get older. No one likes to be singled out and taken out. If there is a way to exit without others knowing about it, such as scheduling extra tuition just after morning break or after lunch, this makes it a lot easier for the student rather than being pulled out in class time when they are at their desks. It is all about being sensitive and thinking about how your struggling students feel.

PART FIVE
FINAL WORD

CHAPTER 11

A final word

Dyslexia describes a student who is developing normally, has had high-quality classroom instruction, has good oral language abilities, and yet has persistent difficulties with reading and writing, especially with decoding and spelling. The essence of dyslexia is that it is unexpected, persistent, and seems out of kilter with the rest of the student's development.

In contrast, many students have reading difficulties for reasons we can understand, such as: they come from disadvantaged home backgrounds, they missed out on appropriate classroom instruction, had difficulties with vision or hearing, or had behaviour or emotional difficulties that interfered with learning. They are usually performing below average in decoding/spelling but also in their ability to understand what they read or listen to. They are said to have mixed difficulties. Many will respond dramatically if they receive appropriate instruction.

There is a final group of struggling readers who can decode and spell but struggle with reading comprehension of material that is at the appropriate level for them. Their difficulties are more in the area of language comprehension. They have fallen behind in vocabulary and general knowledge possibly because they do not read much or may be learning English as another language. A possible solution for them is to read more.

How can parents and teachers help?

Two general approaches

There are two approaches to helping students with dyslexia. One is to work on the areas of difficulty. In other words, improve their decoding and spelling. This means finding a block of time to work in a small group or one-to-one, or arranging cross-age tutoring, peer tutoring, teacher aide help, or specialist help. The other approach is to make 'accommodations' or adjustments in the whole class, such as pairing up the poor reader/speller with a mentor who can help them. Another example of accommodation is to give more time to finish assignments.

Even small changes in teaching can be helpful. Asking students in confidence what they would like you to explain in more detail will help. A 60-second mini-tutorial could help the dyslexic student immensely. There are also classroom opportunities to focus more on decoding skills or spelling, for example, during Big Book reading instruction, where it is possible to demonstrate skills that apply to words in the Big Books they are reading in class, for example, how to break words into their sounds, syllables, or morphemes.

Don't make things worse than they are

One message from the literature is that students with reading difficulties have had a hard time in the past and have become anti-reading. A good suggestion is not to advertise the difficulty. If you want to get help for the student, seek it in confidence. There is a stigma out there, a tendency to write someone off if they have literacy difficulties rather than teach them properly. When you are teaching, for example, take opportunities to explain to the class (and indirectly to the dyslexic reader) how to decode unfamiliar words like sporophyte, explaining that it has a Greek spelling (ph), and showing how to break it into syllables (spor-o-phyte).

We suggest avoid saying, "I'll explain this to you all because I know Ian will appreciate the help". It is best not to embarrass dyslexic students by mentioning them by name in front of a group if it has to do with their reading or spelling, unless it is to say something nice. Instead, we suggest be aware of their needs, and help out quietly without letting the rest of the class know. When marking their essays, perhaps ask them if they want you to focus on spelling or if they want you to focus just on their arguments and ideas. A suggestion is to use a pencil rather than a red pen because it is friendlier when marking.

Reading practice

Be sure to give dyslexic students reading materials that are at the appropriate level of difficulty, and that are not too hard for them to read on their own. Give successful reading experiences. Encourage students to practise the decoding skills they learn, and show them that these skills are useful. Find words in their texts that they have already learned (e.g., silent *e* words) and explain them so they see that they apply in context. Be a model decoder

When you are reading materials to the class, explain what unusual words mean, use the word analysis strategies we have suggested in the book to sound out words, break them into meaningful parts, or break them into syllables to make them easier to pronounce. All these things are designed to keep your students reading and writing. For students with dyslexia, it is all about practice, and this will give them the practice they need.

Concluding comments

Many successful people in our society have dyslexia. It is possible to compensate for these difficulties and still do well. Having dyslexia can range from being mildly annoying to being absolutely frustrating. In this book we have tried to explain different kinds of reading difficulty, including dyslexia, but with a focus on teaching those with dyslexia. As a result, the book is mostly about word decoding and spelling, because these are the proximal causes of difficulty for students with dyslexia, rather than about reading comprehension and the process of writing though we have included some ideas for these areas as well. We hope the ideas are helpful and we would be very interested in your feedback so that we can make improvements for next time.

APPENDICES
RESOURCES

APPENDIX 1

Assessment Measures

Assessment measures in Appendix 1. These measures are all discussed in Chapter 7: Screening for Dyslexia.

Appendix 1A: Burt Word Reading Test
Appendix 1B: Bryant Test of Basic Decoding Skills
Appendix 1C: Alphabet Test (alphabet names and sounds)
Appendix 1D: GKR Phonemic Awareness Test
Appendix 1E: Invented Spelling Test

APPENDIX 1A

Burt Word Reading Test

When giving the Burt Word Reading Test, be sure to follow this procedure:
1. Give the word card to the pupil and say, "This card has some words I think you can read. Let's see which ones you know. Start here and read the words across the card." [Point from word to word, left to right, so the pupil understands what you mean.]
2. The pupil holds onto the special pupil card (see Figure A1.1). Do not let the pupil read from the teacher record sheet (see Figure A1.2).
3. Ask the pupil to start at the beginning of the pupil word card and continue until 10 successive words are read incorrectly. Then say, "Look over the rest of the words and see if you can read more." Sometimes the pupil may recognise another word or more, though this does not often happen. (I remember one pupil could recognise the word *beware* because she recognised it from a "Beware of the dog" sign on her newspaper round.)
4. There is no time limit. Give the pupil ample time to attempt the words.
5. Do not prompt the pupil in any way. Do not ever tell the pupil the correct word. Do not give any clues. Use praise to encourage the pupil, such as "Good boy/girl. Keep going."
6. The word is scored as correct if it is correctly pronounced. The pupil may pronounce the word phonetically, but this will still count as a miscue unless it also sounds correct. For example, the pupil might sound out the word *return* phonetically as *rett-ern*, but the correct pronunciation is *re-turn*, so it is a miscue. If the stress is incorrect, for example, pronouncing *journey* with the stress on the last syllable as in "jer-**nee**", then it is counted as a miscue, since this is not the correct pronunciation. However, be sure to make allowance for children who might have a slightly different way of using stress because of their accent or dialect or have a speech difficulty with certain sounds. If you think they do know the word, give them full credit.

7. Try not to ask the pupil to repeat the word unless you are not sure what the pupil said. In order not to upset the pupil or imply that their first attempt was incorrect, say to the pupil, "I didn't hear what you said for that word. Would you please say it again?"
8. If the pupil reads so quickly you do not have time to record what they say, ask the pupil to slow down, or stop and start reading again more slowly. Go back to the words where you lost track of what the pupil was saying and let the pupil start again.
9. Be sure not to give any clues as to whether the pupil is right or wrong. Do not give any facial expressions that might cue the pupil. If the pupil says, "Is that right?" simply say, "You're doing just fine. Keep going."

Recording the pupil's responses

Complete the personal details at the top of the teacher record sheet before you begin the assessment. Record the pupil's responses unobtrusively, without letting the pupil see what you are doing. For words read correctly, give a tick (√) in the space next to the word. If the pupil miscues, be sure to write down exactly what the pupil says. This can later be analysed to gain some idea of what decoding skills the pupil lacks. If the pupil refuses to make an attempt or is unable to think of something, write DK (don't know) in the space next to the target word. At the end of the assessment, count the number of correct responses and record this in the box in the top right corner of the teacher record sheet.

Interpretation of raw scores: finding the pupil's approximate reading level

In Figure A1.3, to make the raw scores meaningful, the developers of the Burt Word Reading Test have given an indicative estimate of the pupil's reading age for each raw score. The raw scores have been converted to equivalent age bands (EABs). Each age band is based on the age of pupils scoring at one standard error of measurement above and below that mean score. Put another way, for each raw score the age band indicates that this would put the pupil's reading level at about the same level as other pupils in that age range.

In Figure A1.3 the age bands are presented for boys and girls together, as well as separately for boys and girls. This has been done to acknowledge that boys typically do not read as well as girls. In our experience, however, it is better to use the combined boys-and-girls age bands so that you have the same scoring baseline for both boys and girls.

Figure A1.1: Student copy of Burt Word Reading Test

to   is   up   for   big
he   at   one   my   sun

went girl   boys   day   some
his   that   of   an   wet

love   water   no   just   pot
or   now   things   told   sad

carry   village   quickly   nurse   beware
return scramble   twisted   journey   luncheon

known   shelves   explorer   tongue   projecting
terror serious   belief   events   emergency

refrigerator   steadiness   obltain   overwhelmed   universal
nourishment   encyclopaedia commenced   circumstances   fringe

formulate   motionless   trudging   theory   destiny
scarcely   exhausted   labourers   urge   atmosphere

apprehend   binocular   domineer   melodrama   economy
ultimate   reputation   humanity   excessively philosopher

autobiography   contemptuous   terminology   mercenary   glycerine
unique   microscopical   perpetual   efficiency   inrtuential

perambulating   renown   physician   champagne   exorbitant
hypocritical   atrocious   constitutionally   contagion   palpable

melancholy   eccentricity   fatigue   phlegmatic   fallacious
alienate   poignancy   phthisis   ingratiating subtlety

Burt Word Reading Test © Reprinted with permission of New Zealand Council for Educational Research

Appendix 1: Assessment Measures

Figure A1.2 Teacher record sheet for Burt Word Reading Test

Teacher record sheet – the Burt Word Reading Test

Name of student: _____   Number correct: _____
School: _____   Equivalent age band _____
Gender: _____   Norms used (circle one) _____
Year of school: _____   Boys/Girls: Boys and Girls _____
Age: years months _____   Name of assessor: _____
Date of assessment: _____

to	is	up	for	big
he	at	one	my	sun
went	girl	boys	day	some
his	that	of	an	wet
love	water	no	just	pot
or	now	things	told	sad
carry	village	quickly	nurse	beware
return	scramble	twisted	journey	luncheon
known	shelves	explorer	tongue	projecting
terror	serious	belief	events	emergency
refrigerator	steadiness	obtain	overwhelmed	universal
nourishment	encyclopaedia	commenced	circumstances	fringe
formulate	motionless	trudging	theory	destiny
scarcely	exhausted	labourers	urge	atmosphere
apprehend	binocular	domineer	melodrama	economy
ultimate	reputation	humanity	excessively	philosopher
autobiography	contemptuous	terminology	mercenary	glycerine
unique	microscopical	perpetual	efficiency	influential
perambulating	renown	physician	champagne	exorbitant
hypocritical	atrocious	constitutionally	contagion	palpable
melancholy	eccentricity	fatigue	phlegmatic	fallacious
alienate	poignancy	phthisis	ingratiating	subtlety

Figure A1.3: The 6-month age bands for calculating reading age on the Burt Word Reading Test (a suggestion is to find the raw score, then the age band, and take the mid-point of the age band—use the column for boys and girls)

Score	Equivalent Age Bands Boys & Girls	Boys	Girls	Score	Equivalent Age Bands Boys & Girls	Boys	Girls
20	5.10-6.04	6.01-6.07	—	50	8.04-8.10	8.09-9.03	8.01-8.07
21	5.11-6.05	6.02-6.08	—	51	8.05-8.11	8.10-9.04	8.02-8.08
22	6.00-6.06	6.04-6.10	5.09-6.03	52	8.06-9.00	8.11-9.05	8.03-8.09
23	6.01-6.07	6.05-6.11	5.10-6.04	53	8.08-9.02	9.00-9.06	8.04-8.10
24	6.02-6.08	6.05-6.11	5.11-6.05	54	8.09-9.03	9.01-9.07	8.05-8.11
25	6.03-6.09	6.06-7.00	6.00-6.06	55	8.10-9.04	9.02-9.08	8.06-9.00
26	6.04-6.10	6.07-7.01	6.01-6.07	56	8.11-9.05	9.03-9.09	8.07-9.01
27	6.05-6.11	6.08-7.02	6.02-6.08	57	9.01-9.07	9.05-9.11	8.08-9.02
28	6.06-7.00	6.09-7.03	6.04-6.10	58	9.02-9.08	9.06-10.00	8.09-9.03
29	6.07-7.01	6.10-7.04	6.05-6.11	59	9.04-9.10	9.08-10.02	8.11-9.05
30	6.08-7.02	6.11-7.05	6.06-7.00	60	9.06-10.00	9.09-10.03	9.00-9.06
31	6.09-7.03	7.00-7.06	6.07-7.01	61	9.08-10.02	9.11-10.05	9.02-9.08
32	6.10-7.04	7.01-7.07	6.08-7.02	62	9.09-10.03	10.00-10.06	9.03-9.09
33	6.11-7.05	7.02-7.08	6.09-7.03	63	9.11-10.05	10.02-10.08	9.05-9.11
34	7.00-7.06	7.03-7.09	6.10-7.04	64	10.00-10.06	10.04-10.10	9.06-10.00
35	7.01-7.07	7.04-7.10	6.11-7.05	65	10.02-10.08	10.06-11.00	9.08-10.02
36	7.02-7.08	7.05-7.11	7.00-7.06	66	10.03-10.09	10.07-11.01	9.10-10.04
37	7.03-7.09	7.06-8.00	7.01-7.07	67	10.04-10.10	10.09-11.03	10.00-10.06
38	7.04-7.10	7.07-8.01	7.02-7.08	68	10.06-11.00	10.11-11.05	10.02-10.08
39	7.05-7.11	7.08-8.02	7.03-7.09	69	10.07-11.01	11.01-11.07	10.04-10.10
40	7.06-8.00	7.09-8.03	7.04-7.10	70	10.09-11.03	11.03-11.09	10.06-11.00
41	7.07-8.01	7.11-8.05	7.05-7.11	71	10.10-11.04	11.05-11.11	10.07-11.01
42	7.08-8.02	8.00-8.06	7.06-8.00	72	11.00-11.06	11.07-12.01	10.09-11.03
43	7.09-8.03	8.01-8.07	7.07-8.01	73	11.01-11.07	11.09-12.03	10.11-11.05
44	7.10-8.04	8.02-8.08	7.07-8.01	74	11.03-11.09	11.10-12.04	11.00-11.06
45	7.11-8.05	8.03-8.09	7.08-8.02	75	11.05-11.11	12.00-12.06	11.02-11.08
46	8.00-8.06	8.04-8.10	7.09-8.03	76	11.07-12.01	12.02-12.08	11.04-11.10
47	8.01-8.07	8.05-8.11	7.10-8.04	77	11.09-12.03	12.04-12.10	11.06-12.00
48	8.02-8.08	8.06-9.00	7.11-8.05	78	11.11-12.05	12.06-13.00	11.08-12.02
49	8.03-8.09	8.07-9.01	8.00-8.06	79	12.01-12.07	12.09-13.03	11.09-12.03
				80	12.03-12.09	—	12.00-12.06

APPENDIX 1B

Bryant Test of Basic Decoding Skills

Directions

Make a copy of the test for yourself and the student. Give the student copy to the pupil. Ask the pupil to read the words to you, starting with the first column, reading down the column. Then the pupil reads the second column, and then the third column. If the pupil goes too fast for you record responses, ask them to slow down. The student reads the words aloud and you record their answers on your examiner sheet. Explain to the pupil that the words are alien words from outer space and they are not English words. If the pupil tries to turn the words into English words, e.g., says "buf" as "bus" or "butter", stop and explain they are not English words. Put a check mark √ next to the word if it is correct and if incorrect write the incorrect response next to the word. See the pronunciation key below for advice on how the words need to be said. A general rule for beginner readers is to stop after 10 consecutive errors but for older pupils who are having reading difficulties it is helpful to persevere to the end of the test to gather diagnostic information about their ability to decode more difficult words. Chapter 7 gives advice on how to interpret different sections of the test for diagnostic information. The test can also be useful to assess spelling if you give it as a spelling test—it gives diagnostic information on how well the student is breaking words into syllables and sounds for spelling.

Pronunciation Key

1. buf (as in "muff")	26. phune (as in "tune")
2. cos (as in "toss")	27. cho (as in "go")
3. dit (as in "hit")	28. shi (as in "shy")
4. fev (as in "Bev")	29. whe (as in "he")
5. gac (as in "sack")	30. thade (as in "made")
6. huz (as in "buzz")	31. staw (as in "store")
7. jod (as in "cod")	32. plew (as in "flew")
8. kib (as in "rib")	33. fler (as in "her")
9. lek (as in "neck"	34. smar (as in "bar")
10. maz (as in "jazz")	35. blor (as in "floor")
11. nuv (as in "love")	36. cleef (as in "leaf")
12. pof (as in "off")	37. troob (as in "tube")
13. quig (as in "big")	38. spail (as in "mail")
14. rel (as in "bell")	39. groy (as in "boy")
15. san (as in "pan")	40. groaf (as in "loaf")
16. tup (as in "cup")	41. cosnuv (as in cos-nuv)
17. vom (as in "from")	42. relhime (as in rel-hime)
18. wix (as in "six")	43. defev (as in de-fev)
19. yeg (as in "leg")	44. gaction (as in gak-shun)
20. zad (as in "bad")	45. prefute (as in pre-fute)
21. fute (as in "cute")	46. uncabeness (as in un-cabe-ness)
22. yode (as in "code")	47. exyoded (as in ex-yode-ed)
23. bime (as in "time")	48. sanwixable (as in san-wicks-able)
24. nepe (as in "keep")	49. bufkibber (as in buff-kibb-er)
25. cabe (as in "babe")	50. vomazful (as in vom-az-ful)

Appendix 1: Assessment Measures

Alien Words Test

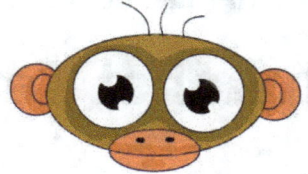

Student Copy

The following words are from an alien language. Can you read them?

buf	fute	cosnuv
cos	yode	relhime
dit	bime	defev
fev	nepe	gaction
gac	cabe	prefute
huz	fune	uncabeness
jod	cho	exyoded
kib	shi	sanwixable
lek	whe	bufkibber
maz	thade	vomazful
nuv	staw	
pof	plew	
quig	fler	
rel	smar	
san	blor	
tup	cleef	
vom	troob	
wix	spail	
yeg	groy	
zad	groaf	
		Total ....../50

Bryant Test of Basic Decoding Skills © Dale Bryant

APPENDIX 1C

Alphabet Test

Instructions

Teacher says: "Look at these letters of the alphabet. Can you read these for me? Can you put your finger on the first letter at the top of the page? What is its name? What sound does it make?" Then move to the next letter and repeat. Be sure that the letters are read left to right across the page. Do this for all the uppercase and lowercase letters.

Scoring of the alphabet test

1. For **names** of letters, accept only the correct names (e.g., C is *cee*).
2. For **sounds**, accept the most common sound (e.g., for C it is *k* and for G it is *g*, as in *got*). If the sound is not known, then you could also ask, 'Can you tell me a word that starts with this sound?' (e.g., *go* for the letter *g*). Either is correct. If the student gives a word that begins with the sound, be sure to record the word.
3. Put a tick in the scoring column if correct, and if incorrect, be sure to record the error.
4. Score out of 26 for names and 26 for sounds.

Student copy of the alphabet test (see below)

Make a copy of this card and give it to the pupil. Ask the pupil to give you the name and sound of each letter, both upper and lower case letters. Do the upper case first because these tend to be easier for them to do.

Score sheet (see below)

The teacher can use this sheet to record responses. Be sure to write down the errors if there are any. For example the pupil might say the name of the letter "g" is /jee/ but the sound is /j/ instead of /g/. The letter "g" can have a /j/ sound but we want its most well-known sound which is /g/ for "goat". Write the total scores for names and sounds,

Appendix 1: Assessment Measures

for upper and lower case, out of 26 at the bottom of the chart. Make a note of letters that will need more instruction, ones the pupil is confused about.

Record the pupil's responses on the scoring sheet (see below).

Student Copy

B	A	I	S	C	
D	F	E	P	T	
L	M	R	Z	J	
U	H	G	W	X	
Q	K	V	Y	N	O
r	o	n	l	m	
y	t	v	k	p	
z	i	a	j	u	
s	h	b	c	g	
w	d	f	x	q	e

Alphabet Test © Reprinted with permission of Tom Nicholson

Score Sheet

Upper case	Names	Sounds	Lower case	Names	Sounds
B			r		
A			o		
I			n		
S			l		
C			m		
D			y		
F			t		
E			v		
P			k		
T			p		
L			z		
M			i		
R			a		
Z			j		
J			u		
U			s		
H			h		
G			b		
W			c		
X			g		
Q			w		
K			d		
V			f		
Y			x		
N			q		
O			e		
Total /26			Total /26		

APPENDIX 1D
GKR Phonemic Awareness Test

GKR Phonemic Awareness Test

Directions: Remember that this is not a reading test. The student does not see the words in the test. You have to read the questions out aloud to the pupil. The test is made up of 6 subtests. Give a practice item before each subtest so the pupil knows what you want h/she to do. A suggested practice word is "cat". For example in subtest 1 on blending, the practice will be to ask the pupil to say each phoneme separately, and then tell you what the word is: Say c-a-t. What word is c-a-t? --- Pupil's answer should be "cat". In subtest 4 segmentation say to the pupil: Say "cat". What are the 3 sounds in "cat"? The pupil should say c-a-t. And so on.

If the pupil has difficulty with the practice item, give the correct answer. Explain what is involved. When you start the real test items, however, do not give any more explanation. Just give supportive comments like "Good boy/girl", "That's good", "OK, let's try another one". Only give corrective feedback for the practice items.

Item Number	Section 1. Blending	Practice: In this task the teacher says the word "cat" slowly, one phoneme at a time and asks the pupil to repeat what she has said: "Say c-a-t. What word is c-a-t?" (answer = "cat")		
		Answer:	Pupil's Response (if incorrect)	
1. "Say n-i-c-e. What word is n-i-c-e?"		nice		
2	t-oo	too		
3	h-e	he		
4	r-a-ke	rake		Subtotal /7 _____
5	t-r-ai-n	train		
6	p-l-a-ne	plane		
7	f-u-nn-y	funny		
Section 2. Deletion of last phoneme		Practice: In this task the teacher says the word normally and then asks the pupil to say the word without its last phoneme: "Say cat. Now say cat without the teh." (answer= "ca")		
		Answer:	Pupil's Response (if incorrect	
8 Say "same". Now say "same" without the (m)		say		
9	me (e)	m		
10	ate (t)	ay		Subtotal /7 _____
11	go (o)	geh		
12	frog (g)	fro		
13	grab (b)	grah		
14	stride (d)	strie		
Section 3. Deletion of first phoneme		Practice: In this task the teacher says the word normally and asks the pupil to say the word without its first phoneme: "Say <u>cat</u>. Now say cat without the "keh". (answer = "at")		
		Answer	Pupil's Response (if incorrect	
15 Say "top". Now say "top' without the (t)		op		
16	gasp (g)	asp		
17	find (f)	ind		Subtotal /7 _____
18	paint (p)	aint		
19	up (u)	p		
20	at (a)	t		
21	so (s)	o		

Appendix 1: Assessment Measures

		Section 4. Phonemic segmentation	Practice: In this task the teacher says the word normally and asks the pupil to say how many phonemes are in the word: "Say cat. What are the 3 sounds in cat?" (answer = keh-a-teh)		
			Answer	Pupil's Response (if incorrect)	Note: Pupil must say the phonemes, not spell the word
	22	Say "no". What are the 2 sounds in "no"	n-o*		*answer is n-o, not "en-oh"
	23	2 – at	a-t		
	24	2 – up	u-p		Subtotal /7
	25	3 – keep	k-ee-p		_____
	26	3 – man	m-a-n		
	27	3 – teeth	t-ee-th		
	28	4 – into	i-n-t-oo		
		Section 5. Substitution of first phoneme	Practice: In this task the teacher says the word normally and asks the pupil to delete the first phoneme and add a new phoneme: "Say cat. Now, instead of keh, start the new word with f." (answer = "fat")		
			Answer	Pupil's Response (if incorrect	
29 Say "ball". Instead of "b" begin a new word with "c"			call		
30		goat b	boat		
31		took c	cook		Subtotal /7
32		fish d	dish		_____
33		two z	zoo		
34		chair p	pair		
35		meat f	feat		

Section 6	Substitution of final phoneme	Answer	Pupil's Response (if incorrect)	Practice: In this task the teacher says the word normally and asked the pupil to delete the last phoneme and add a new phoneme. "Say cat. Now instead of "t", end the word with "p". Answer is "cap"
36	Say park. Instead of "keh", end the word with "t"	part		
37	run (g)	rug		
38	late (m)	lame		
39	mess (n)	men		
40	rope (d)	rode		
41	fame (s)	face		Subtotal /7 _____
42	wet (b)	web		
				Total out of 42 _____

Gough-Kastler-Roper (GKR) Phonemic Awareness Test © Reprinted with permission of Philip Gough

APPENDIX 1E

Invented Spelling Test

This test consists of 18 words. It assesses the extent to which the pupil has the ability to use letter names or sounds to represent all the sounds in words. The value of the test is that you can use the test for diagnostic purposes.

Instructions

Ask the pupil to write their name and the date at the top of a lined piece of paper and then the numbers 1 to 18 down the left side of the paper. If they do not know how to do that, do it for them. We suggest also provide an alphabet chart to help. A copy of the test is below. The pupil does not see this. Explain that you will say the word, say it in a sentence, and say it again. Explain that they are to write each word next to the number they have on the page. Say, "The first word is *fat*. My dog is too *fat. fat*. Write fat next to number 1." Then the teacher moves to the next word on the test list.

Do not help with any of the words and do not correct the spellings. Give only general encouragement. Go slowly. Give time for the pupil to think. If possible, try to complete all 18 words in the task.

Scoring the test

The scoring tries to capture different stages of spelling:

Score = 0, pre-phonemic, using letters but they do not capture the sounds in the word

Score = 1, letters represent at least one sound

Score = 2, letters represent two or more sounds but the spelling does not sound like the actual word

Score = 3, invented spelling where the spelling does sound like the word even though it is not the conventional spelling

Score = 4, correct spelling

For example:

Test word	Miscue	Score
duck	rbotpa	0
duck	d	1
duck	dac	2
duck	duc	3
duck	duck	4

At the bottom of the pupil's spelling sheet, calculate the total score out of 18—this is the total of words spelled correctly. Also calculate the points score that indicates their ability to capture the sounds of the words. This is out of 72 (18 words x 4 points per word).

Teacher Test Sheet

	Say the Word	Say it in a sentence	Say word again
1	fat	My dog is too fat.	fat
2	fill	Please fill my glass	fill
3	lump	He has a lump on his head	lump
4	pop	Don't pop the balloon	pop
5	bank	She put her money in the bank	bank
6	side	He painted the side of the house	side
7	hay	Cows like to eat hay	hay
8	meat	Dogs like to eat meat	meat
9	kick	She likes to kick the ball	kick
10	hot	It was a hot day	hot
11	pack	She put her book in the pack	pack
12	yell	Never yell in the classroom	yell
13	van	Father has a big van	van
14	duck	She gave the duck some bread	duck
15	jail	Robbers go to jail	jail
16	bit	The cat bit her finger	bit
17	cake	The children ate some cake	cake
18	tight	The shoe was too tight	tight

Invented Spelling Test © Reprinted with permission of Jane Prochnow, Bill Tunmer, and James Chapman

APPENDIX 2

Edward Fry's 200 common words, in order of frequency

List 1 1–25	List 2 26–50	List 3 51–75	List 4 76–100	List 5 101–125	List 6 126–150	List 7 151–175	List 8 176–200
the	or	will	number	new	great	put	kind
of	one	up	no	sound	where	end	hard
and	had	other	way	take	help	does	picture
a	by	about	could	only	through	another	again
to	word	out	people	little	much	well	change
in	but	many	my	work	before	large	off
is	not	then	than	know	line	must	play
you	what	them	first	place	right	big	spell
that	all	these	water	year	too	even	air
it	were	so	been	live	mean	such	away
he	we	some	call	me	old	because	animal
was	when	her	who	back	any	turn	house
for	your	would	oil	give	same	here	point
on	can	make	now	most	tell	why	page
are	said	like	find	very	boy	ask	letter
as	there	him	long	after	follow	went	mother
with	use	into	down	thing	came	men	answer
his	an	time	day	our	want	read	found
they	each	has	did	just	show	need	study
I	which	look	get	name	also	land	still
at	she	two	come	good	around	different	learn
be	do	more	made	sentence	farm	home	should
this	how	write	may	man	three	us	world
have	there	go	part	think	small	move	high
from	if	see	over	say	set	try	every

APPENDIX 3

Lesson plans for teaching children with dyslexia to read

These lessons relate to the discussion in Chapter 7: Teaching Children with Dyslexia to Read

Lesson plans

    (a) Lesson plan for short *e* vowel
    (b) Lesson plan for consonant *y*
    (c) Lesson plan for consonant blend *st*
    (d) Lesson plan for long *i* vowel
    (e) Lesson plan for vowel digraph *oa*
    (f) Lesson plan for open and closed syllables

(a) Lesson plan for the short *e* vowel

Aim of the lesson

"By the end of this lesson you will be able to read words with the short *e* vowel, as in *pet*."

Introduction

Suggested introduction: "All words have a least one vowel. Can you remember the names of the five vowels? I will write the vowels on the whiteboard." Write the vowels on the whiteboard, or use magnetic letters. The whiteboard will look something like this:

a   e   i   o   u

Appendix 3: Lesson plans for teaching children with dyslexia to read

Lesson

Suggested lesson: "I have written one vowel in red: *e*. This is the vowel we are going to be learning about today. The *e* makes the sound /ĕ/. Let's say the /ĕ/ sound together.

"If we add the /ĕ/ sound to t (/ĕ/ + /t/) we get /ĕt/. Let's say this new sound together." Write the letters **et** on the board, as shown below, or use magnetic letters. Together read /et/. The whiteboard might look something like this:

```
a   e   i   o   u

        et

        et

        et

        et
```

Either write or place the magnetic letters *b*, *p*, *s*, *g*, *m* and *l* above the *et*. Ask the student to find the letter *s*, then write or place the letter *s* next to the *et*. Together read the word *set*. Ask the student to find the letter *m*, and then place it next to the *et*. Together read the word *met*. Repeat for the other consonants *b*, *p*, *g* and *l*, and any other consonants you might like to include (e.g., *j*, *n*, *v* and *w*).

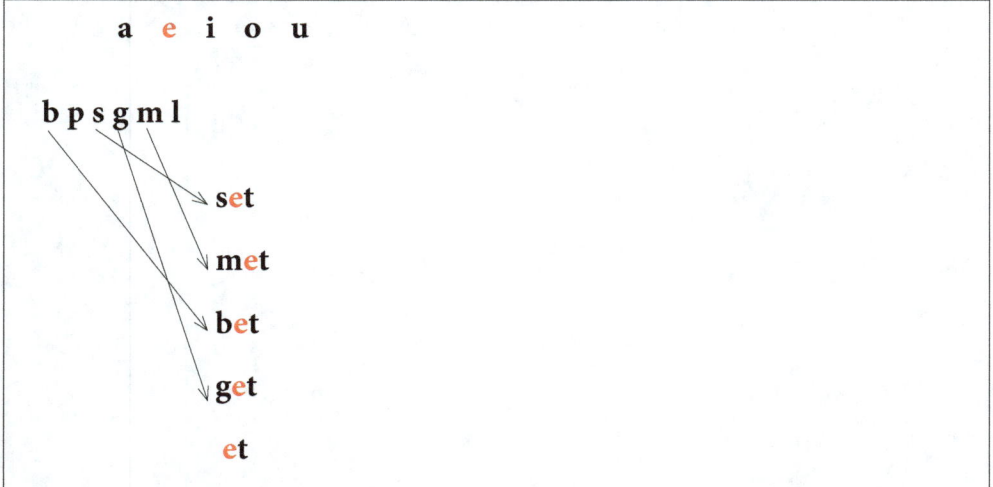

Ask the student to read the words in varying order (e.g,. from *set* to *get*, and then *get* to *set*), and in any order (e.g., *bet*, *set*, *get*, *met*). The words could be put on cards (e.g., *met*) and the student asked to read the words on the cards. Then using a whiteboard marker (or magnetic letters), the student spells the words.

Before concluding the lesson, have the student teach you about the short *e* vowel. This enables you to assess whether the student has grasped what was covered. If there is uncertainty, then short *e* should be either retaught or reviewed in the next lesson.

Remember that students with dyslexia are experiencing decoding difficulties. The assessments showed that Ryan was experiencing difficulty reading words with short *e*. It is likely that students with dyslexia will need more than one lesson on a decoding strategy.

Conclusion

Explain the purpose of the lesson and what was covered. Say something like this: 'Today we have been learning about the short *e* vowel. There are five vowels (*a*, *e*, *i*, *o* and *u*). We have been learning about the short *e*. The short *e* makes an /ĕ/ sound.'

Appendix 3: Lesson plans for teaching children with dyslexia to read

(b) Lesson plan for the consonant *y*

Aim of the lesson

'By the end of this lesson you will be able to read words with the consonant *y*.'

Introduction

Suggested introduction: "There are 21 consonants and 5 vowels, but one consonant is sometimes a consonant and sometimes a vowel. This is the letter *y*. If the letter *y* is at the end of a word it is a vowel, as in *by*, *fly* and *my*. If the letter *y* is at the beginning of a word, as in *yes*, *yellow* and *you*, it is a consonant." Show the student using the whiteboard:

The letter *y*	
vowel	**consonant**
b*y*	*y*es
fl*y*	*y*ell
m*y*	*y*ellow
	*y*ou
	*y*et
	*y*our

The lesson

Suggested lesson: "Today we are focusing on the consonant *y*, but it is important to remember the letter *y* is sometimes a vowel. Write the letter *y* on the whiteboard, both uppercase and lowercase: Y and y. The consonant *y* makes a 'yeh' sound. Let's say the sound together: /y/. Let's say it again: /y/." The following YouTube clip shows how to teach the consonant *y* sound.

http://www.youtube.com/watch?v=lfMCEa1ga-M

"We will now add a sound to the /y/ sound: /y/ and /ee/ = *yee*. Say *yee*. Say it slowly. Stretch it out like *y-eeeee*.

"I will write some words on the whiteboard that start with the letter *y*. We will read them together: *yes*, *yet* and *you*. Let's read again." Then say, "I will point to the words and you can read them."

Consonant *Y y*
yes
yet
you

Ask the student if they can think of other words that start with *y*. Add these to the list on the whiteboard. Practise reading, together and then individually.

Consonant *Y y*

yes	yellow
yet	yell
you	young
year	your
yarn	yard
yesterday	
youth	

Conclusion

Recap what was covered in the lesson: "Today we have learned to read words that start with the consonant *y*. The consonant *y* makes the sound /y/, as in *yet* and *yes*. Look for words that start with *y* when you are reading this week."

Appendix 3: Lesson plans for teaching children with dyslexia to read

(c) Lesson plan for the consonant blend *st*

Aim of the lesson

"Today we are learning to read words that start with the blend *st*."

Introduction

Suggested introduction: "You can read words with the single consonant *s*, like *sat*, *set* and *sit*, and the single consonant *t*, as in *tap*, *tip* and *top*. Well done. Today we are going to learn to read words that have both consonants: *s* + *t*. When we put the two consonants together we call it a consonant blend: /st/."

The lesson

Suggested lesson: "I have written the consonant blend *st* on the whiteboard. First let's say the sound for the letter *s*: /s/. Now let's say the sound for the letter *t*: /t/. Now we will put them together: /st/. We will say the blend slowly: /s-t/. Can you hear both consonants? Each consonant keeps its sound in a blend. This is important to remember. They are blended together, but we can still hear their individual sounds."

```
s + t = st
```

"I have written some words on the whiteboard. Let's read them together. Now you can read on your own. Well done. Notice how the beginning sound for each word is the same: /st/."

```
s + t = st
stub
stab
stop
stag
```

"Here is another list of words. I have taken away the *s* this time. There is no longer a blend at the beginning of the word. Let's read the words."

s + t = st
tub
tab
top
tag

"You will see that an *s* can be added to the beginning of each word to make the /st/ blend. Let's read the words now. Well done."

s + t = st
s + tub = **st**ub
s + tab = **st**ab
s + top = **st**op
s + tag = **st**ag

"Other /st/ blend words include *stay, step, stem, stew, stir, start, stud, story, star, steal* and *steep*."

Conclusion

Review the lesson content. To check that the student does have a good understanding of the *st* blend, have the student 'teach the teacher'. In other words, reverse the roles.

Note: There are many other blends that start with *s* (*sc, sk, sl, sm, sn,* and *sp*). We do not recommend teaching a number of strategies in one lesson. Rather, keep it simple and focus on one strategy at a time. However, if the student is older and grasps the lesson quickly, then more than one blend per lesson can be taught.

(d) Lesson plan for the long vowel sound *i*

Aim of the lesson

"By the end of the lesson you will be able to read words with the long *i* sound (or magic *e* words)."

Introduction

Suggested introduction: "There are five vowels. Which letters are vowels?" Record them on the whiteboard. "Vowels have two sounds. One sound is short and one is long. Today we are learning about the long *i* vowel, but before we learn about the long *i* vowel we will review the short *i* vowel."

The lesson

Suggested lesson: "On the whiteboard I have listed words with a short *i* vowel sound. Let's read the list of words." Point to the whiteboard. "The seven words all have a short *i* vowel sound."

a	e	i	o	u
kit				
bit				
hid				
fin				
spin				
rip				

"Vowels can also be long. A long vowel sounds the same as the name of the letter. So the long *i* vowel sound is /ī/, as in *eye* or *hijack*. To make the short vowel in *kit* into a long vowel, we add *e* to the end of the word. The letter *e* is not pronounced, it is silent. The *e* acts as a marker."

"Some refer to the *e* as bossy *e* or magic *e*. Why is this? Because the *e* makes the vowel say its name. Now that is magic! I will show you how this works so you can use the strategy when you read. I will add *e* to *kit* and our new word is *kite*. Notice that there is only one consonant between *i* and *e*. For the *i* to be long, there can only be one consonant. We will now make all the short vowels long by adding *e* to the end of each word." Together read the list of long *i* vowels.

a e i o u	
short	**long**
kit + e	kite
bit + e	bite
hid + e	hide
fin + e	fine
spin + e	spine
rip + e	ripe
tim + e	time

Conclusion

Suggested conclusion: "Today we learned about the long *i* vowel sound. Let's review what we learned.

- Vowels have two sounds, one short and one long.
- Long vowels say their name (e.g., long vowel *i* is pronounced *eye*).
- The letter *e* acts as a marker. It is sometimes referred to as magic *e* or bossy *e*.
- To make the vowel long, a single consonant comes between the *i* and the letter *e*."

Note: It is likely that a lesson on long vowels will need to be repeated. Vowels present the greatest challenges for readers, particularly readers with dyslexia.

Appendix 3: Lesson plans for teaching children with dyslexia to read

(e) Lesson plan for the vowel digraph *oa*

Introduction

Suggested introduction: "Today we are learning about the vowel digraph *oa*".

The lesson

Suggested lesson: "We have learned that vowels can be short, as in *rid*, or long, as in *ride*. We have learned that long vowels say their name. Can you hear the /ī/ in *ride*? And the /ī/ in *hide*? And the /ī/ in *fine*?

'In English we also have vowel digraphs. Vowel digraphs are two vowels that are grouped together in a word. Words such as *boat*, *coat* and *float* have the vowel digraph *oa*. With vowel digraphs, the first vowel is long (or says its name) and the second vowel is silent."

Put the following on a whiteboard. Magnetic letters or whiteboard markers can be used. Read the words. Ask the student to underline the vowel digraph *oa* in each word.

Vowel digraph: oa	
boat	groan
coat	toast
load	throat
loaf	loan
float	oak

Conclusion

Suggested conclusion: "Today we have worked on the vowel digraph *oa*. When we read words with the vowel digraph *oa*, the *o* is long (so we say its name) and the *a* is silent. Today when you read, write down any words you come across with the *oa* digraph."

(f) Lesson plan for open and closed syllables

Note: This lesson is for students with an understanding of short and long vowels. Teachers may decide to teach one lesson on closed syllables and one lesson on open syllables.

Introduction

Suggested introduction: "Today we are learning about closed and open syllables. A syllable is a unit of speech sound that has a vowel. There may or may not be a consonant before and/or after the vowel. The following unit-of-speech sounds are syllables: *cat*, *at* and *ta*. Some syllables are words like *hat* or *dog*, and some syllables are part of a word such as *hap/py*: *happy*. *Hap* is not a word, but it is a syllable, and *py* is not a word but it is a syllable.

"Today we are learning about two different syllables: closed syllables and open syllables."

Introduce closed syllables first. Note: closed syllables, according to Henry (2010), make up 43 percent of syllables in English. Closed syllables are common in the Anglo-Saxon layer of English and they are the main syllable in Latin roots.

The lesson

Suggested lesson: "Closed syllables are where the single vowel has a consonant after it. In closed syllables the vowel is short. I will write some closed syllables on the whiteboard. Let's read them.

Closed syllables		
at	pet	not
hat	hop	met
it	up	in
pup	fit	add

"Now we will look at words with two syllables where both syllables are closed. First we will underline the vowels. Then we will separate the two syllables. Note that after each vowel there is a single consonant. This makes the vowel short. One way of remembering the syllable is closed is that a consonant or consonants come after the vowel."

Appendix 3: Lesson plans for teaching children with dyslexia to read

Closed syllables	
r<u>a</u>bb<u>i</u>t	r<u>a</u>b/b<u>i</u>t
<u>u</u>ps<u>e</u>t	<u>u</u>p/s<u>e</u>t
k<u>i</u>tt<u>e</u>n	k<u>i</u>t/t<u>e</u>n
n<u>a</u>pk<u>i</u>n	n<u>a</u>p/k<u>i</u>n
<u>i</u>ns<u>e</u>ct	<u>i</u>n/s<u>e</u>ct
c<u>o</u>nt<u>e</u>st	c<u>o</u>n/t<u>e</u>st

"Now we will learn about open syllables. About 32 percent of syllables are open. They are not as common as closed syllables, but they are the second most common. This means that 75 percent of syllables are either open or closed. Open syllables are when a consonant does not follow the vowel in the syllables. The following are open syllables: *he*, *free*, *hi*. You can hear that the vowel is long: it says its name. Let's underline the vowels in the following words. Note that each syllable ends with a vowel."

Open syllables
me
he
hi
free
tree

"Now we will look at two-syllable words where one syllable is open. First we will underline the vowels and break the words into two syllables. Then we will read the words."

Open syllables	
paper	pa/per
open	o/pen
begin	be/gin
student	stu/dent
prefix	pre/fix

"The first syllable in each word is open, so the vowel sound is long. The second syllable is closed, and so the vowel is short. Knowing about closed and open vowels helps us pronounce the syllables.

"Here are some words. Divide the words into syllables and tell me which syllables are closed and which ones are open. Remember to begin by underlining the vowels. They provide an important clue.

- e<u>ve</u>n e/ven [*e-* is an open syllable; *ven* is a closed syllable]
- bedroom bed/room [both syllables are closed]
- photo pho/to [both syllables are open]
- create cre/ate [both syllables are open]
- client cli/ent [*cli-* is an open syllable and *ent* is a closed syllable]
- resistant re/sis/tant [*re-* is an open syllable; *sis* and *tant* are closed syllables]
- provide pro/vide [both syllables are open]
- an an [closed syllable]
- important im/port/ant [all syllables are closed]
- clue clue [an open syllable]."

Conclusion

Suggested conclusion: "Today we have been learning about closed and open syllables." (Note: you may have focused on one of the two syllable types in the lesson.) "Knowing how to break words into syllables and whether they are closed or open helps us to read the words."

APPENDIX 4

Spelling activities

(a) Practice for phonemic awareness – turtle talk
(b) Dot-to-dot phonics
(c) Phonics strips
(d) Sound boxes

(a) Practice for phonemic awareness – turtle talk

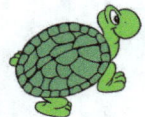

You will need:

- an A3 teacher copy of the turtle talk card (see Figure A4.2)
- copies of the card for pupils
- pencils for the class

The teacher might say: 'Hello class. Today we are practising turtle talk. We are going to break words into their sounds and say them slowly. Remember that a rabbit talks quickly because it runs quickly, and a turtle talks slowly because it walks slowly, so we are going to talk slowly.' Ask pupils to say each word slowly in turtle talk, e.g., f-i-sh. Practice saying the sounds slowly so that pupils can segment the phonemes easily. e.g., f-i-sh, fish, m-o-p, mop, and so on.

Figure A4.2: Illustrations that can be used when teaching phonemic awareness

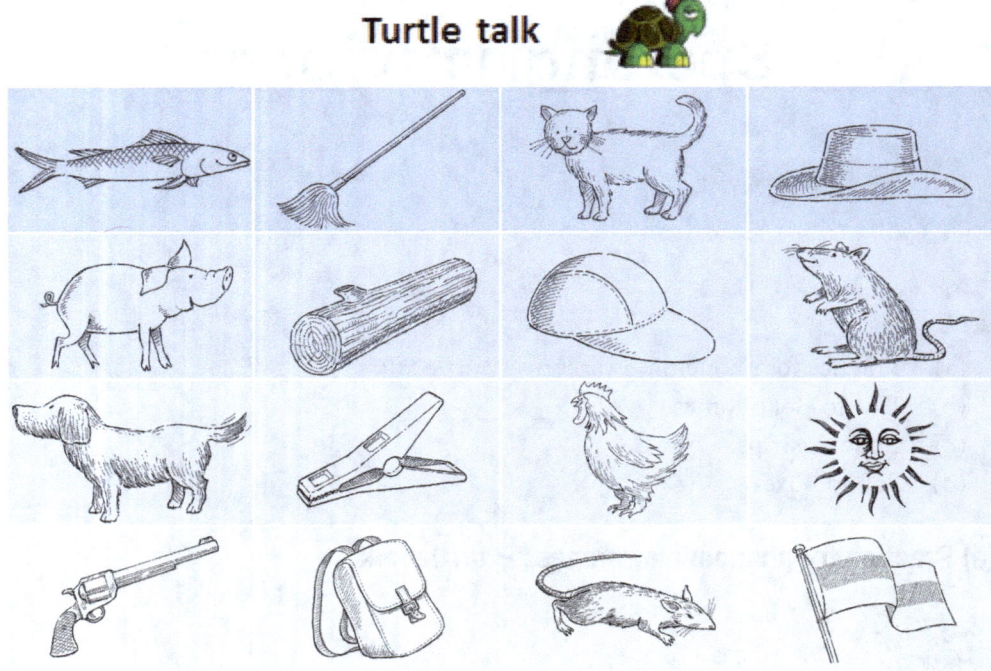

(b) Dot-to-dot phonics

Once pupils are skilled at breaking the spoken words into phonemes, show how to spell the words in the diagram above. First, write the word on the whiteboard, then say the word slowly, pointing to each letter. Ask pupils to say the sounds slowly with you as you point to each letter.

The teacher might say: 'In this activity we are using dots for the sounds in the word we want to spell. Put three dots under the picture of the "log", one for each sound On top of each dot we will write in the letter that goes with that dot. Let me show you.' Teacher writes three dots.

'The first sound in /log/ is? Good, it is /l/. I will write the /l/ sound on the first dot.'

'What is the second sound? (Yes, it is /o/) I will write the /o/ on the second dot.

'Let's say the word slowly /l-o-g/. What is the last sound? (Yes, it is /g/). I will write the last sound.

'Well done. Now we will see if you can spell the words in the turtle talk chart yourself, using dot-to-dot phonics. Write your spellings under each picture. (Teacher gives out copies of Figure A4.2)

Appendix 4: Spelling activities

(c) Phonics strips

You can copy the word lists in Appendix 6 to make your own phonics strips (see example below). Use the lists that have regular spellings—they have been set up so you can make them into phonics strips.

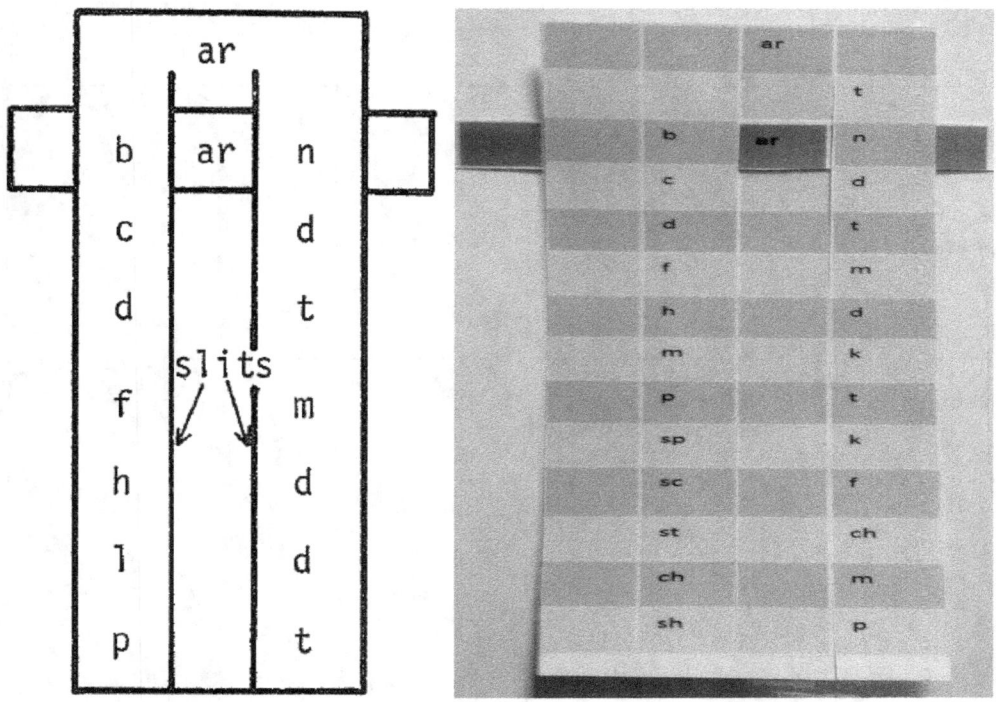

Students can practise reading these patterns, then spelling them.

(d) Sound boxes

Pupils can use sound boxes (see below) to separate out each phoneme before spelling them. Teacher then dictates words from the chart and pupils write the words according to their phonemes, one in each sound box.

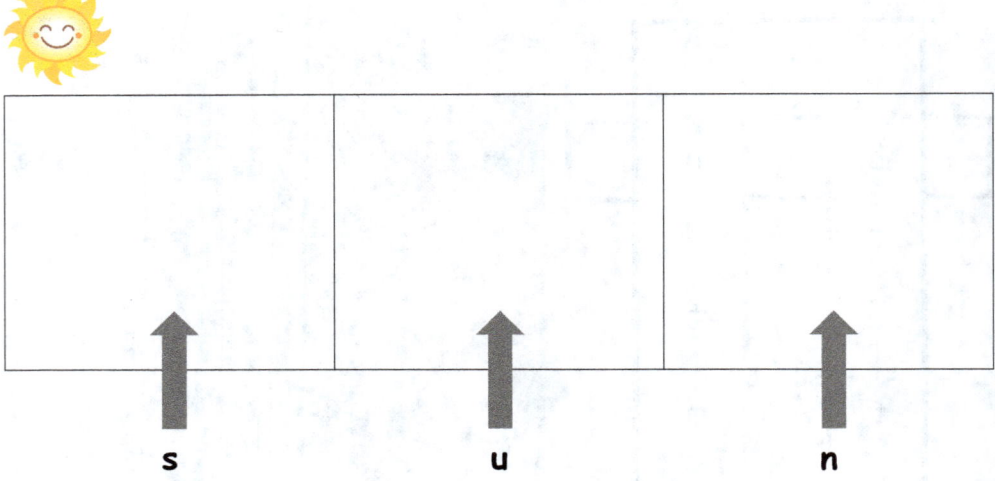

APPENDIX 5

Phonogram charts

Ideas for teaching phonogram patterns
1. Put the phonogram charts on the classroom wall as a reference.
2. Only teach one or two rime patterns at a time. Copy two patterns and make copies for the class. Read the patterns with them and then ask them to fold their page in half while you dictate the words. Have the students check their spellings.
3. Teach them how to spell a key word like *an*, and then show them how to make more words, like *ban* and *can*. Put a dot under each letter and ask your students to say each sound separately and then blend them together.
4. Explain the rule for some of the patterns (e.g., -*ck* is for the /k/ sound at the end of a word after a short vowel, as in *stock*). Explain that it is hard to hear some sounds, like the *n* in *junk*, but it is easier if you spell *jun* and then add a *k*. Explain that it is *ai* at the start or in the middle of a word and *ay* at the end. Explain how the silent *e* rule works in words such as *smoke*.
5. Compare and contrast some spellings, e.g., *ore* and *aw* are both at the end of a word and both spell the same sound /or/.
6. Use sound boxes to spell words (see below). Be sure to explain that there is a box for each sound, not each letter; for example:

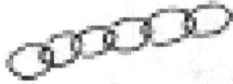

ch		ai	n
t	r	ai	n

7. Ask your students to search for other words in their graded readers that have the same pattern as in the charts (e.g., -*eat* in *heater*).
8. Make a jumble of rime words, and have students sort them into their rimes.
9. Give a spelling test regularly to check that they are using the rime patterns in their spelling.

Chart A

it	ip	ap	in	at	an
it	dip	cap	in	at	an
bit	lip	gap	grin	rat	ban
fit	rip	nap	bin	that	can
hit	sip	rap	pin	cat	fan
sit	tip	slap	chin	fat	man
pit	trip	trap	tin	chat	pan
spit	ship	snap	win	hat	ran
			spin	pat	

uck	ock	ack	ot	ug	op
ruck	dock	back	cot	bug	cop
duck	lock	sack	dot	dug	hop
luck	rock	track	got	hug	pop
tuck	sock	stack	hot	jug	top
stuck	shock	black	not	plug	stop
truck	clock	whack	pot	thug	shop
			spot		

est	ump	ink	unk	ank	ick
best	bump	ink	bunk	bank	brick
nest	dump	link	junk	drank	kick
pest	hump	pink	sunk	sank	lick
rest	jump	rink	drunk	tank	pick
test	lump	sink	trunk	thank	quick
west	pump	wink	skunk	shrank	sick
chest	thump	drink			stick
		think			trick

Appendix 5: Phonogram charts

Chart B

ice	aw	ash
ice rice mice price nice slice	saw raw jaw crawl straw	bash crash dash dash cash flash smash

ake	eat	ing
bake take shake fake snake lake rake	eat beat heat neat seat wheat	king ring sing wing thing string

ay	oke	ill
day play may say tray	woke joke broke smoke choke spoke stroke	ill bill chill fill hill kill pill will spill

ain	ine	ell
pain brain main plain rain strain Spain train	mine pine fine vine line shine nine	bell yell fell shell hell well sell tell

ail	ight	ame
bail rail fail tail jail nail	fight right flight sight night tight knight light	came fame game name tame shame

ale	ide	ore
male whale sale scale pale stale	hide bride ride slide side tide	More store bore core sore wore shore score

APPENDIX 6

A spelling programme to teach Anglo-Saxon vowel spelling patterns

The following programme of spelling is based on spelling information in Jamieson and Jamieson (2003) and Nicholson (2005b). The focus is on vowel sounds because they almost always have multiple ways of spelling them.

Instructions

Assign a list of words each week (the lists are given below), which the students have to revise at home. It is better to give a test on the list when you first hand it out. The students correct any mistakes. Then they take the list away and study it for a follow-up test the next week. This is better than just giving out the list and then testing it the next week. It is called the **test-retest method**.

Each week, explain the spelling pattern in some way. For example, in this list, the /a/ sound in words like *cat* is almost always spelled with the letter *a*.

Show students how to use sound boxes for spelling. Explain that the students, when spelling, should first break each word into its phonemes (or break into syllables first, if the word has more than one syllable) and then spell each syllable phoneme by phoneme.

The lists follow the Anglo-Saxon chart of spellings, starting with short vowel sounds and then moving to long vowel sounds.

Appendix 6: A spelling programme to teach Anglo-Saxon vowel spelling patterns

Overview of spelling programme for vowel sounds
Week

1. The short /a/ sound, as in *at*
2. The short /e/ sound, as in *pet*
3. The short /i/ sound, as in *big*
4. The short /o/ sound, as in *dog*
5. The short /u/ sound, as in *up*
6. The long /ai/ sound as in *bake*, which has three patterns: *a…e*, *ai* and *ay*
7. The long /a/ and ay sound as in *paid* and *pay*
8. The long /e/ sound, as in *bee*
9. The long /e/ sound for e…e pattern: silent e rule
10. The long /i/ sound, as in *like*
11. The long /i/ sound, as in *y* and *igh*
12. The long /o/ sound, as in *go*
13. The long /o/ sound, as in *oa* and *ow*
14. The long /u/ sound as in *cube*, as in u..e and ew
15. The /ar/ sound, as in *car*
16. The /er/ sound, as in *her, sir, fur*
17. The /or/ sound, as in *for*
18. The /or/ sound, as in *launch, claw*
19. The /ow/ sound, as in *cow*
20. The /oi/ sound, as in *toy and oil*
21. The /ue/ sound, as in *broom*
22. The /oo/ sound, as in *good* or *book*

Week 1: Spelling of short /a/ sound, as in *at*

There is basically one way to spell the /a/ sound as in *at*: with an *a*. The exception is *ai*, as in *plait* and *plaid*. Here are some examples of the *a* pattern.

Table A6.1: List of words with short vowel sound — a

	a	
		t
v		n
m		d
r		m
f		n
c		t
r		t
b		t
h		t
c		p
h		m
b		g
c		n
f		t
m		p
s		d

Appendix 6: A spelling programme to teach Anglo-Saxon vowel spelling patterns

Week 2: Spelling of short /e/ sound, as in *pet*

The main pattern for this sound is /e/, as in *pet*, but there is also a set of words that have *ea* as in *bread*, plus some less common spellings. The rule is that *ea* is usually followed by *d*. These patterns are given in the table below.

Table A6.2: List of words with short vowel sound — e as in egg and head

Pattern 1: *e*		Pattern 2: *ea*	
	e		ea
	gg	h	d
b	ll	d	d
p	g	br	d
n	t	r	dy
m	t	br	th
t	n		
h	n		
m	n		
b	d		
r	d		
s	ll		
l	g		
fl	sh		
st	p		
sw	ll		

Table A6.3: Less common spellings for short vowel sound — e as in egg and head

Less common spellings	Words (* remember this one—it is a frequent word)
a	any, many
u	bury (only word like this)
ai/ay	*said (only word like this), says
ie	*friend (only word like this)
ei	leisure, heifer (only words like this)
eo	leopard, jeopardy (only words like this)

Appendix 6: A spelling programme to teach Anglo-Saxon vowel spelling patterns

Week 3: Spelling of short /i/ sound, as in *big*

The main letter pattern for this sound is *i*, but there are some less common spellings such as *y*, as in *myth*.

Table A6.4: List of words with short vowel sound — i as in pig

	i	
		n
b		n
f		t
h		ll
k		ss
f		sh
d		sh
br		ck
cl		p
sp		n
sk		p
st		ck
ch		n
sh		p

Table A6.5: Less common spellings of short vowel sound i as in pig

Less common spellings	Words
y	myth, physics, gypsy
e	pretty, England
u	busy
ui	build
o	women (only word like this)
ie	sieve (only word like this)

Appendix 6: A spelling programme to teach Anglo-Saxon vowel spelling patterns

Week 4: Spelling of short /o/ sound, as in *dog*

The main pattern for this sound is *o*, but there are some less common spellings. These are listed below.

Table A6.6: List of words with short vowel sound — o as in on

	o	
		n
s		cks
fr		g
b		ss
f		g
h		t
m		p
cl		ck
sp		t
bl		ck
st		p
ch		p
sh		ck
str		ng

Other patterns that are less common are given below.

Table A6.7: Less common spellings of o as in on

Less common spellings	Words (* remember this one—it is a frequent word)
a	*was, want, *what, wash, wasp, swan
o...e	gone, scone
ou	cough, trough (only words like this)
au	*because, sausage, Australia
eau	bureaucracy (only word like this)

Appendix 6: A spelling programme to teach Anglo-Saxon vowel spelling patterns

Week 5: Pattern for /u/ sound, as in *up*

The main pattern for this sound is *u*, plus some less common spellings.

Table A6.8: List of words with short vowel sound — u as in up

	u	
		p
b		t
c		t
d		ck
f		n
h		t
n		t
tr		ck
cl		b
st		ck
str		m
sp		n
ch		ck
sl		g

Table A6.9: Less common spellings of u as in up

Less common spellings	Words (* remember this one—it is a frequent word)
o	son, won, money, honey, mother, worry, London, constable
ou	cousin, trouble
o...e	*come, some, done, love
oe	does (only word like this)
oo	blood, flood (only words like this)

Appendix 6: A spelling programme to teach Anglo-Saxon vowel spelling patterns

Week 6: The long /a/ sound as in *bake*, which has three spellings: *a...e*, *ai* and *ay*

Pattern 1: the silent *e* pattern: *a...e*

Table A6.10: List of words with long vowel sound — a as in ate

		a		e	
			t		
	b		k		
	c		m		
	d		z		
	f		m		
	h		t		
	m		k		
	cr		n		
	sp		d		
	sc		l		
	st		k		
	ch		s		
	sh		m		

Week 7: Pattern for *ai* and *ay*

Pattern 2: *ai* at the start or in the middle of a word

This second pattern is the *ai* spelling that goes in the middle of a word like *rain*. The rule is that *ai* is usually followed by *l* or *n*.

Pattern 3: ay—spell *ay* at the end of the word

This third pattern is the *ay* pattern, as in *say*. Notice that we spell *ai* at the end of a word as *ay*. This is because the printers in the old days did not like words to end with the letter *i*, so they did not use *ai*; they used *ay* instead.

Table A6.11: List of words with long vowel sound — a as in aim and say

		ai					ay	
				m	1		d	
	🌧️	r		n	2		s	
		h		l	3		h	
		p		n	4		p	
		b		t	5		sl	
		s		l	6		cl	
		b		l	7		str	
		st		n	8		st	
		br		n	9		tr	
		m		n	10		m	
	🚂	tr		n	11		b	
		ch		n	12		pl	
		n		l	13	🤠	pr	

Appendix 6: A spelling programme to teach Anglo-Saxon vowel spelling patterns

Table A6.12: Less common spellings of long /a/ sound

Less common spellings	Words (* remember this one—it is a frequent word)
ea	steak, great, break
ey	*they, grey, prey, obey
aigh	straight (only one word like this)
ei	vein, rein, abseil
eigh	eight, weigh, sleigh, freight, weight, neighbour
ae	reggae, gaelic (only two like this)
et	ballet, beret, valet, sachet, chalet,

Week 8: The long /e/ sound, as in *bee*, which has three main spellings: *ee*, *ea* and *e...e*

There are three main patterns: *ee*, *ea* and *e...e*.

Pattern 1: *ee* vowel digraph

The rule is that the *ee* spelling is often followed by a *d* or *p*.

Pattern 2: *ea* digraph

A lot of words use *ea* to spell the /ee/ sound.

Table A6.13: List of words with long vowel sound — e as in bee and each

	ee			ea	
		l			t
f		d			s
h		l			t
b		p	b		t
f		d	sn		k
s		d	s		t
sp		d	h		t
st		p	b		d
scr		ch	pl		se
str		t	sp		k
ch		se			
sh		p			

Week 9: Pattern 3: *e...e* pattern: silent *e* rule

Less common is the silent *e* pattern.

Table A6.14: List of words with long vowel sound — e as in Pete

Note that the words get difficult quickly — there are not many easy words with this pattern. You could skip this list for younger pupils.

		e		e
		v		
	P		t	
	th		s	
	g		n	
	extr		m	
	sw		d	
	athl		t	
	concr		t	
	comp		t	
	compl		t	
	sch		m	
	Cr		t	

Table A6.15: Less common spellings of long /e/ sound

Less common spellings	Words (* learn these spellings—they are frequent words)
e	*we, *me, *he, *she, *be
y (after a consonant)	any, baby, many, body, city, family, party, easy, greedy, lucky, funny, carry, happy, jelly, lady, pretty, silly
ey	key, money, honey, donkey, chimney, abbey, hockey, valley, chutney, parsley, trolley, volley
ie	chief, thief, grief, believe, niece, piece, shield, priest
ei	ceiling, receive, seize, caffeine
eo	*people (only one word like this)
ay	quay (only one word like this)
ae	anaemic
oe	phoenix

Appendix 6: A spelling programme to teach Anglo-Saxon vowel spelling patterns

Week 10: The long /i/ sound, as in *like* and *my*, which has one main pattern, *i...e*, and two minor patterns, *y* and *igh*

Pattern 1: *i...e* (silent *e* rule).

This is the split vowel digraph pattern. Sometimes the digraph is not split, as in *pie, lie, tie*.

Table A6.16: List of words with long vowel sound — i as in bike

			i		e	
		b		k		
		b		t		
		k		t		
		d		n		
		t		m		
		h		k		
		m		n		
		cr		m		
		sp		k		
		br		d		
		str		p		
		gr		m		

Week 11: The long /i/ sound, as in *y* and *igh*

Pattern 2: *y*

There is a set of words where the *y* can have the /i/ long vowel sound but it is in the middle or end of a word, not at the start.

Pattern 3: *igh*

There is a set of words where *igh* can have the /i/ long vowel sound but it is in the middle or end of a word, not at the start. The *igh* is usually followed by a *t*. Some of these are given below.

Table A6.17: List of words with long vowel sound — /i/ as in my and high

		y					igh	
	m					h		
	b					r		t
	cr					l		t
	sk					f		t
	wh					kn		t
	st		le			fl		t

Appendix 6: A spelling programme to teach Anglo-Saxon vowel spelling patterns

Table A6.18: Less common spellings of long /i/ sound

Less common spellings	Words (* remember this one—it is a frequent word)
I, i	*I, find, wild, child, pint
ie	pie
eigh	height
eye, -ye	eye, rye, goodbye
ei	either, neither (only words like this)
uy	buy (only one word like this)
ae	maestro

Week 12: The long /o/ sound, as in *bone*, which has three main patterns: *...e*, *oa* and *ow*

Pattern 1: *o...e* (silent *e* rule)

Table A6.19: Lists of words with long vowel sound /o/ as in bone

			o		e	
		b		n		
		c		d		
		c		n		
		d		m		
		l		n		
		h		l		
		m		p		
		n		t		
		r		p		
		t		n		
		v		t		
		w		k		

Appendix 6: A spelling programme to teach Anglo-Saxon vowel spelling patterns

Week 13: The long /o/ sound, as in *oa* and *ow*

Pattern 2: *oa* as in *boat* **Pattern 3:** *ow* as in *tow* (always at end of word)

Table A6.20: Lists of words with long vowel sound /o/ as in coat and tow

		oa					ow	
			k				t	
			t				m	
	b		t				l	
	c		t				bl	
	c		ch				cr	
	r		d				fl	
	g		t				gl	
	l		d				st	
	m		t				sn	
	r		st				sl	
	s		p				kn	
	t		d				thr	
	gr		n					
	br		ch					
	fl		t					

Table A6.21: Less common spellings of /o/ long vowel sound

Less common spellings	Words (* remember this one—it is a frequent word)
o	*go, *no, *so, tomato, potato
ew	sew (only word like this)
oe	toe
ough	though, dough
eo	yeoman (only word like this)
ol	yolk, folk (only words like this)
eau	bureau
oo	brooch

Appendix 6: A spelling programme to teach Anglo-Saxon vowel spelling patterns

Week 14: The long /u/ sound as in *cube* has two main patterns: *u...e* and *ew*

Pattern 1: *u...e* (silent *e* rule)—in middle of word

Pattern 2: *ew*—at end of word

Table A6.22: Lists of words with long vowel sound /u/ as in cute

	u		e			ew	
		t			d		
c		t			f		
d		k			n		
f		m			st		
J		n					
t		b					

Table A6.23: Less common spellings of long /u/ sound

Less common spellings	Words (* remember this one—it is a frequent word)
u	music
eu	neutral
ewe	ewe (only word like this)
eue	queue (only word like this)
eau	beauty
you	*you (only word like this)

Week 15: The /ar/ sound, as in car, has one main pattern: *ar*

Table A6.24: Lists of words with *r*-affected vowel sound /ar/ as in barn

			ar	
				t
		b		n
		c		d
		d		t
		f		m
		h		d
		m		k
		p		t
		sp		k
		sc		f
		st		ch
		ch		m
		sh		p

Table A6.25: Less common spellings of /ar/ sound

Less common spellings	Words
a	fast, last, past
al	half
ear	heart, hearth (only words like this)
er	clerk
au	laugh, aunt, draught

Appendix 6: A spelling programme to teach Anglo-Saxon vowel spelling patterns

Week 16: The /er/ sound, as in her, sir and fur, has three main patterns

Pattern 1: *er*
Pattern 2: *ir*
Pattern 3: *ur*

Table A6.26: Lists of words with *r*-affected vowel sound /er/ as in her, bird, fur

	er			ir			ur	
	h			s			f	
	b	m		b	d		s	f
	g	m		d	t		h	t
	h	b		f	m		b	n
	f	n		f	st		t	n
	h	d		th	st		b	p
	v	b		wh	l		l	ch
				b	th		ch	ch

Table A6.27: Less common spellings of /ir, er, ur/ sound

Less common spellings	Words (* remember this one—it is a very frequent word)
or	work
ear	earth
our	journal, journey (only words like this)
olo	colonel (only word like this)
ere	*were

Week 17: The /or/ sound, as in *corn*, has three main patterns

Pattern 1: *or*

Table A6.28: Lists of words with *r*-affected vowel sound /or/ as in for

		or	
	h		n
	b		n
	c		d
	t		ch
	f		k
	st		k
	m		ning
	p		t
	sp		t
	sc		ch
	st		m
	c		n
	th		n

Appendix 6: A spelling programme to teach Anglo-Saxon vowel spelling patterns

Week 18: *au* **and** *aw*

Pattern 2: *au*

Pattern 3: *aw*

The *aw* pattern is normally at the end of the word and the *au* is in the middle.

Table A6.29: Lists of words with vowel digraphs au and aw for the /or/ sound

		au				aw	
	h		l		r		
	h		nt		p		
	fr		d		l		
	l		nch		l		r
	c		ght		s		
	t		ght		cl		
	s		ce		str		
	l		ndry		dr		
astro	n		t				ful
dino	s		r		pr		n

Table A6.30: Less common spellings of the /or/ sound

Less common spellings	Words (* remember this one—it is a frequent word)
a	*all
al	*talk, walk
ar	war
ore	sore
oor	floor, door, poor
our	four, pour, contour
oar	roar
augh	daughter
ough	brought
ure	sure

Appendix 6: A spelling programme to teach Anglo-Saxon vowel spelling patterns

Week 19: The vowel sound /ow/, as in *cow*, has two main patterns: *ou* and *ow*

Pattern 1: *ou*

Pattern 2: *ow*

The *ow* pattern can be at the end or in the middle of a word. The *ou* pattern is normally in the middle.

Table A6.31: Lists of words with vowel digraph ou and ow for the /ow/ sound

			ou					ow	
				t			c		
		h		se			h		
		sh		t			n		
		c		ch			d		n
		tr		t			g		n
		pr		d			br		n
							cl		n
							dr		n
							fr		n
							gr		l

Table A6.32: Less common spelling of /ow/ sound

Less common spellings	Words
ough	bough, plough (only words like this)

Appendix 6: A spelling programme to teach Anglo-Saxon vowel spelling patterns

Week 20: The /oi/ sound, as in *toy* and *oil*

Pattern 1: *oi* (in the middle of the word)
Pattern 2: *oy* (usually at the end of the word but sometimes at the start or in the middle).

There are no other ways of spelling the /oi/ sound.

Table A6.33: Lists of words with vowel digraphs oi and oy for the /oy/ sound

		oi					oy	
			l				b	
	b		l				j	
	c		n				R	
	j		n				s	
	p		nt				t	
	t		let					ster
	sp		l				r	al
	p		son				l	al
							v	age

Week 21: The /ue/ sound, as in broom

Pattern 1: *oo*

Pattern 2 *ou*

Pattern 3: *ew*

Pattern 4: *ue*

The *ew* and *ue* patterns are normally only at the end of a word.

Table A6.34: Lists of words with vowel digraphs oo, ou, and ue for the /oo/ sound as in moo

oo			ou		ue	
t			s	p	bl	
b			gr	p	tr	
z					cl	
m	n		ew		gl	
r	m	cr			s	
r	f	dr			fl	
s	n	fl				
t	th	gr				
f	d	scr				
br	m					
sw	p					

Appendix 6: A spelling programme to teach Anglo-Saxon vowel spelling patterns

Table A6.35: Less common spellings of the /ue/ sound

Less common spellings	Words (* remember this one—it is a frequent word)
oo...e	choose
o	*do, *who, *to
o...e	move, lose
wo	*two (only word like this)
oe	shoe, canoe (only words like this)
ough	through (only word like this)
u	truth
ui	juice, suit
eu	sleuth

Week 22: The /oo/ sound, as in *good* or *book*

The main pattern is *oo*.

Table A6.36: Lists of words with the vowel digraph oo for the /oo/ sound as in book

		oo	
	b		k
	c		k
	l		k
	h		k
	t		k
	f		t
	s		t
	g		d
	w		d
	cr		k
	br		k
	st		d

Table A6.37: Less common spellings for the /oo sound as in book

Less common spellings	Words (* remember this one—it is a frequent word)
u	put, pull, bull, full, push, bush
ou	*could, *would, *should (we think these are the only words with this spelling of /oo/)

APPENDIX 7

Examples of individual spelling tutoring

Summary of individual spelling lessons:

1. Silent *e* rule
2. *r-* and *l-* affected vowels
3. Vowel digraphs: *ai - ay*
4. Latin spellings: *-ian, -ion*
5. Greek spellings: *ch, ph, y*

1. Silent *e* rule

Today we're learning about the silent *e* rule
Can you remember the five vowels? The first one is?
"*a*"
Next one?
e
Next one?
i
Next one?
o
Last one?
u
Good job
We're doing the *a* first – it has two sounds, long and short. Do you know the short sound for *a*?
a
Good
Do you know the long sound for *a*?
"ay"
Good job
I'm going to give you some words to read to me. What is this? (writes "at")
"at"
Good
What is this? (writes "ate")
(pause)
This is the silent e (points to *e* at end of word) – we don't sound it out - it tells us what is happening to the vowel before it (draws an arrow from the *e* to the *a*) What sound is this? (points to the *a* in "ate")
"ah" – I mean "ay"
Yes it sounds like the long vowel "ay"
What does the word say? (points to "ate")
"ate"
Good job. Now let's see if you can spell "at"
(pupil writes "at")
Well done. Now can you spell "ate"?
(pupil spells "at", pauses, then adds the silent *e*)
Well done!
Can we do one more example?
OK
Let's do this one (writes "plan")
What does that say?
"plan"
Good. What happens if we add *e* at the end? (writes "plane")
(pause)
Remember that the silent *e* makes the vowel before it say its name
"plane"
Good job, well done. Now let's see if you can spell "plan"
(pupil writes "plan")
Well done. Now can you spell "plane"?
(pupil spells "plan", then adds the silent *e*)
Good job!

Appendix 7: Examples of individual spelling tutoring

2. *r*- and *l*-affected vowels

Today I'm going to teach you the *r*- and *l*-affected vowels. First we will write the vowels. Can you tell me how to pronounce their names? (writes a, o, e, i, u)
(pupil says the names of the vowels)
Good job. Now I am going to write the vowels with an r after them. This changes their sound (writes ar, or, er, ir, ur). When we write "a" and then "ll" after it, this changes the "a" sound as well. Can you tell me the sounds of these spelling patterns ?
Teacher writes: ar, or, ar, ar, ar, all
 (pause – student does not say anything)
Let me help you – er, ir, ur have the same sound "er". And "all" is pronounced "orl". Now can you tell me again what the sounds are?
ar, or, er, ir, ur, all
Well done. Now I want you to spell some words that have these patterns. Let's do the ar sound first, spell "arm"
(student spells it)
(teacher then asks to spell ark, dark, shark, star)
Great, well done. Can you underline the "ar" in these words for me?
(student underlines them)
Here is another word, "for" – can you spell it for me?
(pupil writes "for")
Great, now can you spell "her"
(pupil writes "hir")
Close. The "er" sound can be written three ways which make it hard to know which way to spell the word. For example, we spell "her" this way but we spell "sir" this way and 'fur this way. It's the same sound each time but each time we spell the words in a different way. Now let's see if you can spell a word with "all" in it – can you spell "ball"?
Pupil writes "ball"
Great. Before we finish can you tell me the sounds of the patterns again? (Teacher points to ar, or, er, ir, ur, all). Well done. Thank you.

3. vowel digraphs *ai-ay*

Today we're going to learn about vowel digraphs. Can you tell me what they are?
(pause)
They're two vowels that when you put them together make one sound. Today we're going to talk about the vowel digraphs *ai* and *ay*. (Teacher writes the heading "vowel digraphs" at top of whiteboard, then writes the headings "ai" and "ay" in two different columns) Do you know what their sounds are?
"ay"
Very good, ai and ay have the same sound but they are spelled differently, aren't they?
Yes
So can you give me a word that has an *ai* in it?
(pause)
How about this one? (writes "mail" in the "ai" column)
Mail
And this one? (writes "tray" in the "ay" column)
Trail
Is it "trail"? Have a look at the end – it sounds like "ay"
Tray
Very good
And this one? (writes "play" in the "ay" column)
Play
And this? (writes "trail" in the "ai" column)
Trail
And this? (writes "say" in the "ay" column)
Say
Can you underline all the *ai* and *ay* sounds for me?
(she underlines all the *ai* and *ay* patterns)
Can you see the difference between this column and this column?
Yes
What?
Same spelling?
They are similar spellings but slightly different, ai is in the middle of the word and *ay* is usually ...
Last?
Yes, at the end of the word. The reason is that there are very few words in English that end in "i". So when the "ai" sound is in the middle of the word it is spelled *ai* and when you hear the "ai" sound at the end of the word it is spelled *ay*. Does that make sense?
Yes
Can you tell me one more time, so *ai* and *ay*, what is the difference?
(pause)
"ai" is usually ...
Middle
And "ay" is usually ...
End
Very good, well done

Appendix 7: Examples of individual spelling tutoring

4. Latin spellings *-ian, -ion*

Today we're going to talk about Latin words. You can always tell a Latin word because it will often have a special beginning called a prefix or an ending called a suffix that you can add to the word. This makes the word longer but it also changes its meaning as well. Today we will look at two endings. This one is *-ion* (teacher writes *-ion* in one column) and this one is *-ian* (teacher writes *-ian* in another column). Now what I will do is write this word in this column (teacher writes "state"). Can you read that for me?
State
Now I'm going to add *-ion* (teacher adds *-ion*). I'll take off the *e* at the end of "state" because we do not need it any more (Teacher does not tell the student the reason in this lesson but the reason is that the "i" in "ion" will tell the reader that the vowel before it is a long sound so the *e* is not needed). Can you read that for me?
Statin
Let's have a closer look. When we add *-ion*, you can see the "t" and "i" go together. In Latin words, when this happens, it makes the "sh" sound
Station?
Yes, that's it. Is there a station near where you live, a railway station?
(pause)
Is there a petrol station?
Yes
Great. Now let's look at this column. What is this word here? (teacher writes "magic")
Magic
What's magic?
People do magic, play magic
Yes, they do tricks, pull rabbits out of hats, that sort of thing. Now if I add *-ian*, remember that when "c" and "i" go together they make a "sh" sound, what have I written now?
Magikan
Remember that "ci" says "sh"?
Magician
Yes, that's it. Now I'll write another word in the *-ion* column (teacher writes "note). What does that say?
Note
Now I'll add *-ion*.
(student does not say anything)
It says "notion". Now I'll write another word in the *-ian* column (teacher writes "electric"). What does that say?
Electris
Let's have a closer look. That says "electric". It has a "c" at the end to make a /k/ sound. Now I'll add *-ian*. What does the word say now?
Electran
Remember that when the "ci" are together they say "sh" - it says "electrician"
Electrician
Great. Did you know that when you spell *-ian* at the end of the word it means someone who does something — in this column a magician does magic—but in this column the words don't do something, like "station" doesn't do anything, it just stands there, and we spell it with *-ion*. Interesting, eh? That will help you when you are not sure whether to spell *-ion* or *-ian*.

5. Greek spellings—ch, ph, y

Today we are looking at Greek words and how to spell them. A lot of words in English come from the Greek language. It's easy to tell a Greek word because it has a particular spelling. A lot of words spell "ch" for the /ch/ sound like in cheese – and what else?
Chicken?
Yes, but "ch" in a Greek word stands for another sound altogether, it makes a new sound /k/. Here is a Greek word with the "ch" making a /k/ sound. Can you read that? (Teacher writes "school")
School?
Yes, notice that the "ch" has a /k/ sound in "school". Can you underline the "ch" in school?
(student underlines the "ch")
Here's another Greek spelling (teacher writes "ph"). What is the sound of "ph"?
/f/
Yes, it has a /f/ sound. When you see a "ph" spelling, you know it's a Greek word. Let's look at this word (teacher writes "phone"). Can you read that?
Phone
That's great. Can you tell me the last part of the word?
(student pauses)
I can help here - after the "ph", the rest of the word says "own".
Sometimes the letter "y" in the middle of a word can have an "i" or "ie" sound. Then you know it is a Greek word, like this word (writes "gym") can you read that?
Gym
Yes, it's interesting that we spell the word "gym" with a "g" – a lot of words spell the /j/ sound with a "g" because there is a rule that you can use the "g" for /j/ and you can use a "c" for the /s/ sound if it they are followed by an e, i, or y. The word "gym" is short for "gymnasium". A gymnasium is where you play sports.
The "y" in a Greek word can also have an "ie" sound like in these words (teacher writes "type", "cycle" and "style". Can you read these words?
(student reads "cycle" as "kycle")
This word (points to "cycle" says /sycle/), like in "bicycle". There is that rule when "c" is followed by a "y" is has a /s/ sound. Now let's see if you can spell the words without looking at them (teacher dictates "school", "phone", "gym, "type", "cycle", and "style")

APPENDIX 8

Lesson plans combining Big Book reading and explicit phonics to help with spelling

Big Books are enlarged texts you can read to the whole class where they can see all the words. This could be print or digital display such as a smartboard. The lessons make use of four different Big Books.

Summary of focus rule, book and book level

Rule	Book	Level of book
Silent *e* rule	The Hole in the King's Sock (Ready to Read)	Level 15; Orange; 6-6.5 years
Consonant blends	Keep Trying (Ready to Read)	Level 6; Yellow; 5.5-6 years
r- and *l-* affected vowels	Who Likes Greedy Cat (Ready to Read)	Level 4; Red; 5-5.5 years
Vowel digraph *oo, ou*	Magnetic Max (Gilt Edge)	Level 14; Green; 6 year o d
Syllable breaking	Firefighter Fred's Busy Day (Gilt Edge)	Level 19; Purple; 7-7.5 years

Introduction
1. Focus: Silent e rule
2. Story: *The Hole in the King's Sock* (Level 15, Orange, 6-6.5 year level)

Teacher (T): Hello, we are going to learn a rule which is called the silent e rule, and then read the story about the King who found a hole in his sock.
T: Do you know what a vowel is? In English, we have 5 letters with vowel sounds and each letter stands for two sounds, one long and one short. First of all, the 5 vowels are written as: a, e, i, o, u and sometimes y is also included as well. The sounds of the vowels usually change when there is an e at the end of the word, and we call this the silent e rule. (Then recap that the short sounds are the actual sounds of the letters and the long sounds are the names of the letters).

Lesson: (using whiteboard)
T: The silent e rule for *a_e* means that when you see the word spelled *ate* it says "ate"- the special e makes the vowel says its name. (Teacher draws arrow) I am going to underline the vowels.

a t e

T: Remember, the letter e is silent in "ate", and this e is going to make the other vowel "ay" say its name. Let's say this word together.
T: Well done! Let's have a look at some other examples on the whiteboard.

Short vowel	Long vowel
mat	mate
hat	hate
pet	Pete
pin	pine
cop	cope
cut	cute

T: Let's have a look at these words from the story - you are going to see them in the story later.

came	gave	made
wove	stitched	dough
knit	knitting	wriggled
gold	learn	thread

Students look at the word as a whole first, sounding them out if they do not know the word. They repeat and read the words 2 times.

came: c-a-me (silent e)   gave: g-a-ve (silent e)
made: m-a-de (silent e)   wove: w-o-ve (silent e) past tense of weave
stitched: st-i-tch-ed (tch ="ch" sound)   d-ough: irregular word
knit: kn-i-t (silent k)   knitting: kn-i-tt-i-ng
wriggled: wr-i-gg-l-ed (silent w)   g-o-l-d
l-ear-n   th-r-ea-d

Activity: Turtle Talk (researcher selects 5-6 words from chart above)
The students listen to the phonemes of the words provided by the researcher e.g., "m-ay-deh" and they have to point out the correct word on the whiteboard. Pupils get a chance to Turtle Talk and say the word and the teacher has to guess what it is.

The teacher explains the silent e rule again when reading words from the story that had the silent e pattern - *came, gave, made, wove*. The word *dough* from the story is an irregular word. The -tch in *stitched* has the ch sound because ch is spelled tch after a short vowel sound. Explain that *knit* and *knitting* both have a silent k; *wriggled* has a silent w.
T: Great, I am going to read you the story of *The Hole in the King's Sock*, and I am going to ask you some questions about what happened in the story afterwards. Before we start, what are socks? Yes, they are covers we put on our feet. Where do you buy your socks from?
Pupils say: the warehouse, the supermarket, two-dollar shop.
T: Well, we will see what happens to the King's sock. Now, please listen carefully to the story (during the reading, encourage students to predict what might happen next).
Comprehension questions (orally)
1. What was the King's problem?
2. Did he find a solution? What was that?
3. Did it work? If not, why did it not work?
4. Was the problem solved at the end?

Appendix 8: Lesson plans combining Big Book reading and explicit phonics to help with spelling

Consonant blends

Focus
Phonics rule: Consonant Blends
Big Book story: *Keep Trying* (Level 6, Yellow, 5.5-6 year level)
T: The blend "bl" (writes bl on board) stands for two sounds "b" and "l"....like the first two sounds you can hear in "**bl**ue". Let's try another one, the blend sw stands for two sounds? What do you think they are? Yes..."s" and "w" like in "**sw**im".
T: Now, we are going to learn more blends before reading our story *Keep Trying*.

Lesson:
T: Look at this Blends Chart that I have made up:

| br | bl | cr | dr | fl |
| gr | pl | sw | sp | tr |

Let's read the blends in each box – what two phonemes does this blend stand for? (s = students)
S: "bl"...
T: Can you tell me any words that start with "bl"?
S: "blue", "blog"
T: Good. I'll write those down.
Note: students are to sound out each consonant blend with other examples provided by the teacher and class.
T: The story we are going to read today is *Keep Trying*. How did you feel when you had to learn something new? Like riding a bike, learning to swim? Did anyone one help you? *Keep Trying* is about a little boy who learned new things. Before we start reading the story, I would like you all to have a look at these words from the story that are on the whiteboard. Let's see if you can sound them out and know the meanings of them.

can't   could   couldn't
climb   **sk**ate   **sk**ipping
keep   **tr**ying   catch
swim

They follow the teacher and read each sound
They read the words 2 times – the teacher breaks up the sounds as in the chart below and points out features like silent e, irregular verb:

can't : c-a-n-t (irregular word- means cannot)   climb: c-l-i-m-b
keep: k-ee-p   skate: s-k-a-te
 (silent e)
skipping: s-k-i-p-p-i-ng   trying: t-r-y-i-ng
swim: s-w-i-m   catch: c-a-tch
could: c-oul-d (irregular verb)   c-oul-d-n'-t-could not (irregular verb)

Activity: Turtle talk (the teacher writes 5-8 words from list above)
Teacher does Turtle Talk. Students listen to the sounds of the words provided by the teacher, and they point out the correct answer on the whiteboard. For example, the teacher says, "c-a-tch" and pupils say which word it is on the board. Pupils get a chance to Turtle Talk and say the word. For example, the teacher asks the class to choose a word from the list and say it slowly and the teacher will guess the word.

The teacher briefly explains the contractions "can't" and "couldn't".

T: Great, I am going to read you the story now, and afterwards I am going to ask you some questions about what happened in the story. So, please listen carefully.
(During the reading, encourage students to predict what might happen next).
Comprehension questions (Orally)
1. Can you remember the new skills that the little boy learnt in the story? (riding a bike, swimming, skating, catching a ball, climbing a tree).
2. Did anyone help the little boy? (yes) Who? (Father) What did father say to him? (keep trying)
3. There's a skill that the father couldn't do. What was it? (skipping)
4. What's the message of the story? If you want to learn a new skill, what do you need to do?
    (keep trying and you can do it).

r- and l-affected vowels

Focus: Phonics rules -- r- and l-affected vowels Big Book story - *What Does Greedy Cat Like?* (Level 4; Red; 5-5.5 year level) Recap: T: Last week we talked about the sounds "ar", "er", "ir", "or", "ur" where the letter r changes the vowel sound to make a new sound. Like "ar" in "car" and "dark"; "or" in "for" and "pork"; "er" in "her" and "mother"; "ir" in "first" and "thirst"; "ur" in "fur" and "surf" (Teacher writes the words on the whiteboard and underlines all the r-affected vowels).
Lesson: l-affected vowels Teacher: Today we are going to learn about adding -ll after the five vowels. (Whiteboard) Teacher writes words with the *-all* pattern T: The *–al* has an "or" sound in words like "all", "ball", "wall", "mall". It also has an "or" sound in words like "walk" and "chalk" T: Can anyone tell me other words with *al* making the "or" sound? S: "call", "fall", "hall", "tall", "stall" Note to teacher: Other l-affected vowels (e.g., -ell) do not change their sounds the way the –al does Teacher writes words with –el pattern and explains *-el* has an "el" sound like in the words "bell", "sell", "tell", and "fell". Can you tell me a word that has the *–el* pattern? (smell, well, yell, elk) Teacher explains *-il* has a sound like "il" in the words ill, bill, hill, kill and mill. Can you think of a word that has the *–il* pattern? (pill, chill, will, still, milk) Teacher explains *-ol* has a sound like "ol" in the words doll, toll, roll, poll. Can you think of a word that has the *–ol* pattern? (troll, stroll, scroll) Teacher explains *-ul* has a sound like "ul" in the words dull, gull and cull. Can you tell me a word that has *–ul* pattern? (skull, mull, bulk) Note to teacher: Meanings of the words are also explained to the students while learning the sounds.

Turtle talk activity:
T: Now I will write some words from the Big Book story and some other words as well and we will do some turtle talk.
Teacher: let's say each word slowly and I will point to the phonemes as we read
Teacher: Let's look at each word and I will underline the "r" and "l" patterns. What do I underline in "ball"? I will underline some other patterns as well. Let's say these patterns when I point to them

b-all ("orl")	d-oll ("oll")	c-a-ke ("ake")
b-ell ("ell")	s-k-ull ("ull")	d-i-nn-er ("er")
p-ill ("ill")	ch-ee-se ("ch")	n-o-t ("not")

Appendix 8: Lesson plans combining Big Book reading and explicit phonics to help with spelling

T: Let's read the story about Greedy Cat one more time.
T: Good!
T: Do you remember what kind of food Greedy Cat likes the most in the story that starts with the digraph /ch/?
S: Cheese, chips, chocolate….
T: Good

Vowel digraphs – oo and ou

Focus: Phonics rule: vowel digraph *oo* and *ou* Big Book story-*Magnetic Max* (Level 14; Green; 6-year-old level)

Lesson: vowel digraphs *oo* and *ou*
T: We are going to learn the sounds for these vowel digraphs: writes *oo* and *ou*.
 	
T: We are looking at this digraph (points to *oo*) first. It has two sounds. The main sound is "oo" as in "book". The second sound is "ue" as in "moon".
 	
The next vowel digraph is *ou* (points to *ou*). It also has two sounds. The first sound is "ow" as in "out". Another sound is "ue" as in "you". This is the same as the second sound of the "oo" digraph.
 	
Activity1
T: Does the *oo* in this chart (points to *oo*) sound like "oo" or "ue"? (teacher writes the words on the whiteboard, pupils read the words, and then with teacher help choose the correct sound for each word)
   oo - "oo"   oo - "ue"
cook   spoon
took   school
roof   rook
good
 	
Activity 2
 	
   ou - "ow"   ou - "ue"
mouse   soup
house   group
count   you
 	
Phonemic awareness (Turtle Talk)
T: Let's look at words from the Big Book that have the *ou* and *oo* patterns and some other words as well
Teacher writes the words on the whiteboard. Pupils and teacher use Turtle Talk to stretch out the sounds of the words while the teacher points to each phoneme, e.g., "l-oo-keh-deh", "looked"
street   odd
l**oo**ked
our   amazing   flew
paper   morning   **ou**t
time   think   magnet
c**oo**kie   pocket   skateboard
tree   park   dog
 	
R: Today we are reading about Magnetic Max. Look at the picture on the cover. Max and his magnet are hiding in a tree. What is Magnetic Max up to? Let's read the story together and find out

Syllable breaking

Teaching focus:
1. Phonics strategy - Syllable breaking for CVC/CVC words
2. Big Book – *Firefighter Fred's Busy Day* (Level 19; Purple; 7-7.5 year level)

Lesson: Syllable breaking CVC/CVC
Today, we are going to learn how to read longer words. We can break them into small chunks...we call it syllable breaking. Remember, when we speak, we speak in syllables. Words are made up of one or more syllables. Like the word "rabbit"...there are 2 syllables.... (Teacher claps hands to show the students... "rab"..(clap).... "bit"..(clap)---2 syllables. Now, listening carefully....how many syllables can you hear in "robot"? We can clap our hands and find out. ("ro"...(clap)..."bot"...(clap))---2 syllables (Good work!) Remember, every syllable has a vowel sound. I am going to write this word on the whiteboard and show you how to do syllable breaking.

T: (writes *rabbit* on whiteboard) How many vowels are there?
S: Two
T: Good work (puts a tick on top of each vowel sound)

```
    √              √
r   a   b  |  b    i   t
c   v   c  |  c    v   c
```

T: There is a rule for splitting a word like "rabbit". The rule is that if there are two consonants after the first vowel, you split the two consonants in the middle: "rab"-"bit". You can see that "rabbit" has a consonant-vowel-consonant pattern "cvc/cvc"
(Teacher writes cvc under each syllable)
T: When you see the cvc pattern you know that the vowel has its short sound. This cvc pattern is called a closed syllable because it makes the vowel says its short sound. By spelling the word with cvc for "rab" and cvc for "bit" the reader knows that the two vowels have their short sound.

```
r   a   b  /  b    i   t
```

Activity:
Let's have a look at another word. See if you can divide the word into syllables.

```
r   u   b    b    i   s   h
```

T: Do you remember what do you need to do first?
S: Tick all the vowels.
T: Excellent. Two vowel sounds = Two syllables

```
    √              √
r   u   b    b    i   s   h
```

T: Then, what shall we do next?
S: um.....draw a line in the middle....??
T: Whereabouts in the middle? Between which two letters?
S: B and B
T: Great!

```
    √              √
r   u   b   /   b    i   s   h
```

T: Now, we break this word into two small chunks. Can you say the first part? "rub" - then "bish", can you put them together and say it like a word?
S: "rub-bish"
T: Very good

Let's try few more words that are in the story we are going to read.
Syllable breaking and turtle talk – saying the phonemes in the word slowly
rescue (res/cue)
pickle (pic/kle)
cleaning (clea/ning)
vegetables (ve/gee/tay/bles)
squashy (squash/y)
****
T: We are also learning the use of the contracted words today with some of the words in the story. What contracted means is that we leave out some letters and replace them with an apostrophe. For example, when we are writing the word "can't" the apostrophe replaces "no"...it is actually the short form of "cannot". Let's have a look at the list here.

can't	cannot
we're	we are
I'm	I am
it's	it is
I'll	I will

T: Let's read the story together.

Note: Lesson plans are from Tse 2011, Tse & Nicholson, 2014

APPENDIX 9

Questionnaire for Students

How do you feel?	Agree 🙂	Sometimes 😐	Disagree ☹️
1 I enjoy school			
2 I get enough time to copy things down			
3 My teacher often praises me			
4 I get help with my spelling			
5 My teacher thinks I am good at things			
6 I am as important as everybody else in the class			
7 My ideas are as good as everybody else's in the class			
8 I get told off for bad spelling			
9 I get told off for bad handwriting			
10 I often avoid words I can't spell when I am writing			
11 My work is often put on show where everyone can see it			
12 I have time to finish my written work in class			
13 I have time to write my homework down			
14 I have the right equipment for lessons			
15 I think I spend twice as much time on my homework as other people in my class			

Accessing the curriculum	Usually	Sometimes	Never
16 I work with a partner who writes down my ideas			
17 Teachers repeat instructions I have forgotten			
18 Teachers read important information out to the whole class			
19 Teachers take marks off if I make spelling mistakes			
20 There are helpful things for me to use in class, like bookmarks, word mats, a special dictionary, etc.			
21 Teachers give me writing frames/ graphic organisers to help me with my writing			
22 I use special software on the school computer to help me with my writing.			
23 I know that I don't have to read out loud in class unless I want to			
24 I am doing the best school work I can			
25 I am happy at school most of the time			
26 I worry a lot about school			
27 I am proud of my work			
28 One thing that really helps me is			
29 One thing I really hate is			

Note: From Coffield, Riddick, Barmby and O'Neill, 2008, p. 368

References

A conversation with Henry Winkler kicks off the West family 40th anniversary speaker series. (2010). *Benchmark News*, Summer, 3.

Adams, M. J. (1990). *Beginning to read: Thinking and learning about print*. Cambridge, MA: MIT Press.

Al Otaiba, S. A., & Fuchs, D. (2006). Who are the young children for whom best practices in reading are ineffective? *Journal of Learning Disabilities, 39*, 414–431.

Allington, R. L. (1977). If they don't read much, how they ever gonna get good? *Journal of Reading, 21*, 57–61,

Allington, R. L. (2013). What really matters when working with struggling readers. *The Reading Teacher, 66*(7), 520–530.

Allington, R. L., & Gabriel, R. E. (2012, March). Every child every day. *Educational Leadership, 69*(6), 10–15.

Bandura, A. (1993). Perceived self-efficacy in cognitive development and functioning. *Educational Psychologist, 28*(2), 117–148.

Barton, S. M. (2003). Classroom accommodations for students with dyslexia. *Learning Disabilities Journal, 13*(1), 10–14.

Bennett, T. (2009). Strategies and characteristics of one-to-one literacy tutors. *Reading Forum, 24*(1), 27–33.

Bishop, D. V. (2007). Curing dyslexia and attention-deficit hyperactivity disorder by training motor coordination: Miracle or myth? *Journal of Paediatrics and Child Health, 43*, 653–655.

Block, C. C., & Parris, S. R. (Eds.). (2008). *Comprehension instruction: Research-based best practices* (2nd ed.). New York, NY: Guilford Press.

Block, C. C., & Pressley, M. (2003). Best practices in literacy instruction. In L. M. Morrow, L. B. Gambrell, & M. Pressley (Eds.), *Best practices in literacy instruction* (2nd ed., pp. 111–126). New York NY: Guilford Press.

Block, C. C., & Pressley, M. (2007). Best practices in teaching comprehension. In L. B. Gambrell, L. M. Morrow, M. Pressley (Eds.), *Best practices in literacy instruction* (3rd ed., pp. 220–242). New York, NY: Guilford Press.

Borgia, L., & Owles, C. (2011). Terrific teaching tips. *Illinois Reading Council Journal, 39*(3), 50–54.

Bourassa, D. C., & Treiman, R. (2003). Spelling in children with dyslexia: Analyses from the Treiman-Bourassa early spelling test. *Scientific Studies of Reading, 7*(4), 309–337.

Bourassa, D. C., & Treiman, R. (2006). Use of morphology in spelling by children with dyslexia and typically developing children. *Memory and Cognition, 34*(3), 703-714.

British Dyslexia Association. (2006). *Achieving dyslexia-friendly schools resource pack* (5th ed.). Retrieved from http://www.bdadyslexia.org.uk

Brown, R. (2002). Straddling two worlds: Self-directed comprehension instruction for middle schoolers. In C. C. Block & M. Pressley (Eds.), *Comprehension instruction: Research-based best practices* (pp. 337-350). New York, NY: Guilford Press.

Bryant, D. (1975). *Bryant Test of Basic Decoding Skills*. New York, NY: Teachers College Press.

Bryant, P. (2002). Children's thoughts about reading and spelling. *Scientific Studies of Reading, 6*(2), 199-216.

Bryant, P., Nunes, T., & Snaith, R. (2000). Children learn an untaught rule of spelling. *Nature, 143*(6766), 157.

Calfee, R. C. (1983). The mind of the dyslexic. *Annals of Dyslexia, 33*(1), 7-28.

Calfee, R. C. (1984). Applying cognitive psychology to educational practice: The mind of the reading teacher. *Annals of Dyslexia, 34*, 219-240.

Calfee, R. C., & Associates. (1984). *The book: Components of reading instruction.* Unpublished manuscript: School of Education, Stanford University.

Calfee, R. C., & Patrick, C. L. (1995). *Teach our children well*. Stanford, CA: Stanford Portable Book Series, Stanford Alumni Association.

Cassar, M., Treiman, R., & Moats, L. (2005). How do the spellings of children with dyslexia compare with those of non-dyslexic children? *Reading and Writing, 18*(1), 27-49.

Castles, A., & Coltheart, M. (1996). Cognitive correlates of developmental surface dyslexia: A single case study. *Cognitive Neuropsychology, 13*, 25-50.

Chambliss, M., & Calfee, R. C. (1998). *Textbooks for learning: Nurturing children's minds*. Malden, MA: Blackwell.

Chard, D. J., Ketterlin-Geller, L. R., Baker, S. K., Doabler, C., & Apichatabutra, C. (2009). Repeated reading interventions for students with learning disabilities: Status of the evidence. *Exceptional Children, 75*(3), 263-281.

Clay, M. M. (1987). Learning to be learning disabled. *New Zealand Journal of Educational Studies, 22*, 155-173.

Clay, M. M. (1993). *Reading Recovery: A guidebook for teachers in training*. Auckland: Heinemann.

Clay, M. M. (2000). *Running records for classroom teachers*. Portsmouth, NH: Heinemann.

Clay, M. M. (2005). *An observation survey of early reading achievement*. Portsmouth, NH: Heinemann.

Clay, M. M. (2013). *An observation survey of early literacy achievement* (3rd ed.). Auckland: Heinemann.

Clay, M. M., & Imlach, R. H. (1971). Juncture, pitch, and stress as reading behavior variables. *Journal of Verbal Learning and Verbal Behavior, 10*, 133-139.

Coffield, M., Riddick, B., Barmby, P., & O'Neill, J. (2008). Dyslexia friendly primary schools: What can we learn from asking the pupils? In G. Reid, A. Fawcett, F. Manis, & L. Siegel (Eds.). *The Sage handbook of dyslexia* (pp. 356-368). London, UK: Sage Publications.

Coltheart, M., & McArthur, G. (2012). Neuroscience, education, and educational efficacy research. In S. Della Sala & M. Anderson (Eds.), *Neuroscience in education: The good, the bad, and the ugly* (pp. 215-229). Oxford, UK: Oxford University Press.

References

Corballis, M. (2011). *Pieces of mind.* Auckland: University of Auckland Press.

Crist, P. J., & Smith, P. W. (2008). Teacher to teacher: What one activity would you recommend to teach high school students to spell? *The English Journal, 97*(4), 19.

Darr, C., McDowall, S., Feral, H., Twist, J., & Watson, V. (2008). *Progressive Achievement Test.* Wellington: New Zealand Council for Educational Research.

Dunn, L. M., & Dunn, D. M. (2007a). *Picture Peabody Vocabulary Test* (4th ed.). Minneapolis, MN: Pearson Assessments.

Dunn, L. M., Dunn, D. M., Styles, B., & Sewell, J. (2007b). *The British Picture Vocabulary Scale* (3rd ed.) London, UK: NFER-Nelson.

Dymock, S. (2007). Comprehension strategy instruction: Teaching narrative text structure. *The Reading Teacher, 61,* 161–167.

Dymock, S., & Nicholson, T. (2007). *Teaching text structures: A key to nonfiction reading success.* New York, NY: Scholastic.

Dymock, S. & Nicholson, T. (2010). "High 5!" strategies to enhance comprehension of expository text. *The Reading Teacher, 64,* 166–178.

Dymock, S., & Nicholson, T. (2012). *Teaching reading comprehension: The what, the how, the why.* Wellington: NZCER Press.

Dymock, S. J., & Nicholson, T. (2013). *Dyslexia decoded. What it is, what it isn't, and what you can do about it.* Wellington: Dunmore Press.

Edwards, J. (1994). *The scars of dyslexia.* New York, NY: Cassell.

Ehri, L. C. (1987). Learning to read and spell words. *Journal of Reading Behavior, 19,* 5–31.

Ehri, L. C. (2005). Learning to read words: Theory, findings, and issues. *Scientific Studies of Reading, 9,* 167–188.

Ehri, L. C. (2013). Orthographic mapping in the acquisition of sight word reading, spelling memory, and vocabulary learning. *Scientific Studies of Reading, 17,* 1–17.

Ehri, L. C., Nunes, S. R., Stahl, S. A., & Willows, D. M. (2001). Systematic phonics instruction helps students learn to read. *Review of Educational Research, 71*(3), 393–447.

Eissa, M. (2010). Behavioral and emotional problems associated with dyslexia in adolescence. *Current Psychiatry, 17*(1), 17–25.

Elbro, C. (1999). Dyslexia: Core difficulties, variability, and causes. In J. Oakhill & R. Beard (Eds.), *Reading development and the teaching of reading* (pp. 131–156). Oxford, UK: Blackwell.

Eldridge, J. L. (2005). Foundations of fluency: An exploration. *Reading Psychology, 26,* 161–181.

Eldridge, J. L., Reutzel, D. R., & Hollingsworth, P. M. (1996). Comparing the effectiveness of two oral reading practices: Round robin reading and the shared book experience. *Journal of Literacy Research, 28*(2), 201–225.

Elley, W., Ferral, H., & Watson, V. (2011). *Supplementary Tests of Achievement in Reading (STAR).* Wellington: NZCER Press.

Elliott, J. G. (2005, December). The dyslexia debate: More heat than light? *Literacy Today,* 8.

Elliott, J. G. (2006). Dyslexia: Diagnoses, debates, and diatribes. *Education Canada, 46*(2), 14–17.

Elliott, J. G., & Grigorenko, E. L. (2014). *The dyslexia debate.* Cambridge, UK: Cambridge University Press.

Evans, M. A., & Saint-Aubin, J. (2013). Vocabulary acquisition without adult explanations in repeated shared book reading: An eye movement study. *Journal of Educational Psychology, 105*(3), 596–608.

Foorman, B. R., Francis, D. J., Shaywitz, S. E., Shaywitz, B. A., & Fletcher, J. M. (1997). The case for early reading intervention. In B. A. Blachman (Ed.), *Foundations of reading acquisition and dyslexia: Implications for early intervention* (pp. 243-264). Mahwah, NJ: Erlbaum.

Frank, R., & Livingston, K. E. (2002). *The secret life of the dyslexic child*. Princeton, NJ: Philip Lief Group.

Fry, E. (2000). *Dr. Fry's 1000 instant words*. Westminster, CA: Teacher Created Materials.

Garan, E. M., & De Voogd, G. (2008). The benefits of sustained silent reading: Scientific research and common sense converge. *The Reading Teacher, 62*(4), 336-344.

Gentry, J. R. (2000). A retrospective on invented spelling and a forward look. *The Reading Teacher, 54*(3), 318-332.

Gilmore, A., Croft, C., & Reid, N. (1981). *Burt Word Reading Test*. Wellington: New Zealand Council for Educational Research

GL Assessment. (2012). *York Assessment of Reading Comprehension (YARC)*. Melbourne, VIC: Author.

Goswami, U. (n.d.). *Beginning reading acquisition in different languages: A psycholinguistic grain size framework*. Center for Neuroscience, Faculty of Education, University of Cambridge.

Goswami, U. (2009). *Learning difficulties: Future challenges*. London, UK: Government Office for Science.

Goswami, U. (2012). Principles of learning, implications for teaching? Cognitive neuroscience and the classroom. In S. Della Sala & M. Anderson (Eds.), *Neuroscience in education: The good, the bad, and the ugly* (pp. 47-57). Oxford, UK: Oxford University Press.

Gough, P. B. (1993). The beginning of decoding. *Reading and Writing, 5*(2), 181-192.

Gough, P. B. (1996). How children learn to read and why they fail. *Annals of Dyslexia, 46*, 3-20.

Gough, P. B., & Hillinger, M. L. (1980). Learning to read: An unnatural act. *Bulletin of the Orton Society, 30*, 179-186.

Gough, P. B., Hoover, W. A., & Peterson, C. L. (1996). Some observations on a simple view of reading. In C. Cornoldi & J. Oakhill (Eds.), *Reading comprehension difficulties* (pp. 1-13). Mahwah, NJ: Erlbaum.

Gough, P. B., Juel, C., & Griffith, P. L. (1992). Reading, spelling, and the orthographic cipher. In P. B. Gough, L. C. Ehri, & R. Treiman (Eds.), *Reading acquisition*. Hillsdale, NJ: Erlbaum.

Gough, P. B., & Lee, C. H. (2007). A step toward early phonemic awareness: The effects of turtle talk training. *Psychologia, 50*, 54-66.

Gough, P. B., & Tunmer, W. E. (1986). Decoding, reading, and reading disability. *Remedial and Special Education, 7*, 6-10.

Gough, P. B., & Walsh, M. A. (1991). Chinese, phoenicians, and the orthographic cipher of English. In S. A. Brady & D. P. Shankweiler (Eds.), *Phonological processes in literacy: A tribute to Isabelle I. Liberman* (pp. 199-209). Hillsdale, NJ: Erlbaum.

Graves, M. F., Juel, C., & Graves, B. B. (2004). *Teaching reading in the 21st century* (3rd ed.). Boston, MA: Pearson.

Greaney, K. (2000). *Vowel phonograms*. Unpublished manuscript, Institute of Education, Massey University, Palmerston North.

Gresham, F. M., & Vellutino, F. R. (2010). What is the role of intelligence in the identification of specific learning disabilities?: Issues and clarifications. *Learning Disabilities Research & Practice, 25*(4), 194-206.

Grigorenko, E. L. (2012). Genetic sciences for developmentalists: An example of reading ability and disability. In S. Della Sala & M. Anderson (Eds.), *Neuroscience in education: The good, the bad, and the ugly* (pp. 47-57). Oxford, UK: Oxford University Press.

References

Hamill, D. D., & Larsen, S. C. (2009). *TOWL 4: Test of Written Language*. Austin, TX: Pro-Ed.

Harley, T. (2010). *Talking the talk*. Hove, East Sussex: Psychology Press.

Handler, S. M., & Fierson, W. M. (2010). The joint technical report: Learning disabilities, dyslexia, and vision. *Pediatrics, 127*(3), E818–E856.

Hattie, J. (2009). *Visible learning: A synthesis of over 800 meta-analyses relating to achievement*. London, UK: Routledge.

Henry, M. K. (2010). *Unlocking literacy: Effective decoding and spelling instruction* (2nd ed.). Baltimore, MD: Paul H. Brookes.

Hilden, K., & Jones, J. (2012).Traditional spelling lists: Old habits are hard to break. *Reading Today*, June/July, 19–21.

Howard-Jones, P. A. (2011). From brain scan to lesson plan. *The Psychologist, 24*(2),110–113.

Hresko, W. P., Herron, P. K., Peak, P. R., & Hicks, D. L. (2012). *TEWL 3: Test of Early Written Language*. Austin, TX: Pro-Ed.

Hudson, R., Pullen, P., Lane, H. B., & Torgesen, J. K. (2009). The complex nature of reading fluency: A multidimensional view. *Reading and Writing Quarterly, 25*(1), 4–32.

Hughes, L. E., & Wilkins, A. (2000). Typography in children's reading schemes may be suboptimal: Evidence from measures of reading rate. *Journal of Research in Reading, 23*(3), 314–324.

Hurry, J., Nunes, T., Bryant, P., Pretzlik, U., Parker, M., Curno, T., & Midgely, L. (2005). Transforming research on morphology into teacher practice. *Research Papers in Education, 20*(2), 187–206.

Jamieson, C., & Jamieson, J. (2003). *Spelling. Manual for testing and teaching English*. London, UK: Whurr.

Iversen, S., & Tunmer, W. E. (1993). Phonological processing skills and the Reading Recovery program. *Journal of Educational Psychology, 85*(1), 112–126.

Johnston, F. R. (2000/2001). Spelling exceptions: Problems or possibilities? *The Reading Teacher, 54*(4), 372–378.

Joseph, L. M. (1999). Word boxes help children with learning disabilities identify and spell words. *The Reading Teacher, 52*, 348–356.

Judge, S. (2013). Longitudinal predictors of reading achievement among at-risk children. *Journal of Children and Poverty, 19*(1), 1–19.

Juel, C. (1988). Learning to read and write: A longitudinal study of 54 children from first through fourth grades. *Journal of Educational Psychology, 80*(4), 437–447.

Juel, C. (1994). *Learning to read and write in one elementary school*. New York, NY: Springer-Verlag.

Juel, C. (1996). What makes literacy tutoring effective? *Reading Research Quarterly, 31*, 268–289.

Juel, C., Griffith, P. L., & Gough, P. B. (1986). Acquisition of literacy: A longitudinal study of children in first and second grade. *Journal of Educational Psychology, 78*, 243–255.

Kessler, B., & Treiman, R. (2003). Is English spelling chaotic? Misconceptions concerning its irregularity. *Reading Psychology, 24*, 267–289.

Krafnik, A. J., Flowers, D. L., Luetje, M. M., Napoliello, E. M., & Eden, G. F. (2014). An investigation into the origin of anatomical differences in dyslexia. *Journal of Neuroscience, 34*(3), 901–908. doi: 10.1523/JNEUROSCI.2092-13.2013

LaBerge, D., & Samuels, J. (1974). Toward a theory of automatic information processing in reading. *Cognitive Psychology, 6*, 293–323.

McLachlan, C., Nicholson, T., Fielding-Barnsley, R., Mercer, L., & Ohi, S. (2013) *Literacy in early childhood and primary: Issues, challenges, solutions*. Melbourne, VIC: Cambridge University Press.

McIntosh, R. D., & Ritchie, S. J. (2012). Rose tinted? The use of coloured filters to treat reading difficulties. In S. Della Sala & M. Anderson (Eds.), *Neuroscience in education: The good, the bad, and the ugly* (pp. 230–243). Oxford, UK: Oxford University Press.

McNeill, B., & Kirk, C. (2014). Theoretical beliefs and instructional practices used for teaching spelling in elementary classrooms. *Reading and Writing, 27*, 534–555.

Marston, D. (1996). A comparison of inclusion only, pull-out only, and combined service models for students with mild disabilities. *Journal of Special Education, 30*, 121–132.

Martin, F., & Pratt, C. (2001). *Nonword Reading Test*. Melbourne: ACER Press.

Meyer, B. J. F., & Rice, G. E. (1994). The structure of text. In P. D. Pearson, R. Barr, M. L. Kamil, & P. Mosenthall (Eds.), *Handbook of reading research* (Vol. 1, pp. 319–351). New York, NY: Longman.

Miller, G. A. (1956). The magical number seven, plus or minus two: Some limits on our capacity for processing information. *Psychological Review, 63*, 81–97.

Millward, B. (2004). How has dyslexia affected me? In T. R. Miles (Ed.), *Dyslexia and stress* (2nd ed., pp. 139–142). London, UK: Whurr.

Milne, D. (2014). *Teaching the brain: The new science of education*. Huntington Beach, CA: Junior Learning.

Ministry of Education. (1996). *Dancing with the pen*. Wellington: Learning Media.

Ministry of Education. (2007). *The New Zealand curriculum for English-medium teaching and learning in Years 1–13*. Wellington: Learning Media.

Ministry of Education. (2008). *About dyslexia*. Wellington: Author.

Moats, L. C. (2000). *Speech to print: Language essentials for teachers*. Baltimore, MD: Paul H. Brookes.

Morgan, W. P. (1896). A case of congenital word blindness. *British Medical Journal, 2*, 1378.

Morris, R. (2012). *Teacher professional development and learning survey*. Auckland: Unpublished manuscript.

Mortimore, T., & Dupree, J. (2008). *Dyslexia-friendly practice in the secondary classroom*. Exeter, UK: Learning Matters.

Murray, B. A., & Steinen, N. (2011). Word map/ping: How understanding spelling improves spelling power. *Intervention in School and Clinic, 46*, 299–304.

National Institute of Child Health and Human Development. (2000a). *Report of the National Reading Panel: Teaching children to read: An evidence-based assessment of the scientific research literature on reading and its implications for reading instruction* (NIH Publication No. 00- 4769). Washington, DC: U.S. Government Printing Office.

National Institute of Child Health and Human Development [Producer]. (2000b). *When stars read* [Video]. Washington, DC: Author. https://www.youtube.com/watch?v=3blqhClqGNo

Neale, M. D., McKay, M. F., & Barnard, J. (1999). *Neale Analysis of Reading Ability* (3rd ed.). Melbourne, VIC: Australian Council for Educational Research.

New Zealand Council for Educational Research. (2010). *Progressive Achievement Test: Listening comprehension*. Wellington: NZCER Press.

Nicholson, T. (1986). Taking the guesswork out of reading. *Set: Research Information for Teachers, 2*, Item 14.

Nicholson, T. (1997). Closing the gap on reading failure: Social background, phonemic awareness and learning to read. In B. Blachman (Ed.), *Foundations of reading acquisition and dyslexia* (pp. 381–407). Hillsdale, NJ: Erlbaum.

References

Nicholson, T. (1999). Family, literacy and society. In G. B. Thompson & T. Nicholson (Eds.), *Learning to read: Beyond phonics and whole language* (pp. 1–24). New York, NY: Teachers College Press.

Nicholson, T. (2000). *Reading the writing on the wall: Debates, challenges and opportunities in the teaching of reading*. Melbourne, VIC: Thomson.

Nicholson, T. (2003). Risk factors in learning to read, and what to do about them. In B. Foorman (Ed.), *Preventing and remediating reading difficulties: Bringing science to scale* (pp. 165–196). Timonium, MD: York Press.

Nicholson, T. (2005a). *At the cutting edge: The importance of phonemic awareness in learning to read and spell*. Wellington: New Zealand Council for Educational Research.

Nicholson, T. (2005b). *Phonics handbook*. Chichester, UK: Wiley.

Nicholson, T. (2008). Achieving equity for Maori children in reading by 2020. *New Zealand Annual Review of Education, 18*, 159–182. Retrieved from http://www.victoria.ac.nz/NZAROE

Nicholson, T. (2014). Academic achievement and behavior. In P. Garner (Ed.), *Sage handbook of emotional and behavioural difficulties* (2nd ed., pp. 177–188). London, UK: Sage.

Nicholson, T., & Dymock, S. (2010). *Teaching reading vocabulary*. Wellington: NZCER Press.

Nicholson, T., & Dymock, S. (2011). Matthew effects and reading interventions. *Perspectives on Language and Literacy, 37*, 28–33.

Nicholson, T., & Gallienne, G. (1995). Struggletown versus Middletown: A comparison of reading achievement among pupils from different social classes. *New Zealand Journal of Educational Studies, 30*, 15–24.

Northway, N. (2003). Predicting the continued use of overlays in school children: A comparison of the developmental eye movement test and the rate of reading test. *Ophthalmic and Physiological Optics, 23*, 457–464.

O'Connor, R., White, A., & Swanson, L. (2007). Repeated reading versus continuous reading: Influences on reading fluency and comprehension. *Exceptional Children, 74*(1), 31–46.

O'Connor, R. E., Swanson, H. L., & Geraghty, C. (2010). Improvement in reading rate under independent and difficult text levels: Influences on word and comprehension skills. *Journal of Educational Psychology, 102*, 1–19.

Ouellette, G., & Sénéchal, M. (2008). Pathways to literacy: A study of invented spelling and its role in learning to read. *Scientific Studies of Reading, 12*(2), 195–219.

Ouellette, G., Sénéchal, M., & Haley, H. (2013). Guided children's invented spelling: A gateway into literacy. *Journal of Experimental Education, 81*(2), 261–279.

Palomo-Alvarez, C., & Puell, M. (2013). Effects of wearing yellow spectacles on visual skills, reading speed, and visual symptoms in children with reading difficulties. *Graefe's Archive of Clinical & Experimental Opthalmology, 251*(3), 945–951.

Panagos, R. J., & Dubois, D. C. (1999). Career self-efficacy development and students with learning disabilities. *Learning Disabilities Research & Practice, 14*, 25–34.

Parkin, C., & Parkin, C. (2011). *PROBE 2: Reading comprehension assessment kit*. Wellington: Triune Initiatives.

Pashler, H., McDaniel, M., Rohrer, D., Bjork, R. (2008). Learning styles: Concepts and evidence. *Psychological Science in the Public Interest, 9*(3), 105–119.

Pikulski, J. J., & Chard, D. J. (2005). Fluency: Bridge between decoding and comprehension. *The Reading Teacher, 59*, 570–519.

Polacco, P. (1998). *Thank you, Mr Falker*. New York, NY: Philomel Books.

Pressley, M. (2002). Comprehension strategies instruction. In C. Block & M. Pressley (Eds.), *Comprehension instruction: Research based practices* (pp. 11–27). New York, NY: Guilford Press.

Pressley, M. (2008). What the future of reading research could be. In C. C. Block & S. R. Parris (Eds.), *Comprehension instruction: Research-based best practices* (2nd ed., pp. 391–413). New York, NY: Guilford Press.

Prochnow, J.E., Tunmer, W.E., & Chapman, J.W. (2013). A longitudinal investigation of the influence of literacy-related skills, reading self-perceptions, and inattentive behaviours on the development of literacy learning difficulties. *International Journal of Disability, Development, and Education, 60,* 185–207.

Prochnow J. E., Tunmer, W. E., Chapman, J. W., & Greaney, K. (2001). A longitudinal study of early literacy achievement and gender. *New Zealand Journal of Educational Studies, 36*(2), 221–236.

Read, C., & Treiman, R. (2013). Children's invented spelling: What have we learned in forty years? In M. Piatelli-Palmarini & R. C. Berwick (Eds.), *Rich languages from poor inputs* (pp. 197–211). New York, NY: Oxford University Press.

Reid, G. (2010). *Dyslexia* (2nd ed.). London, UK: Continuum.

Reutzel, D. R., Petscher, Y., & Spichtig, A. N. (2008). Exploring the value added of a guided silent reading intervention: Effects on struggling third grade readers' achievement. *Journal of Educational Research, 105*(6), 404–415.

Reynolds, D., & Nicolson, R. (2008). Letters to the Editor: Comment on 'Curing dyslexia and attention deficit hyperactivity disorder by training motor coordination: Miracle or myth?' *Journal of Paediatrics and Child Psychology, 44,* 521.

Riddell, S. (2009). Social justice, equality, and inclusion in Scottish education. *Discourse: Studies in the Cultural Politics of Education, 30*(3), 283–296.

Riddick, B. (1996). *Living with dyslexia.* London, UK: Routledge.

Riddick , B. (2006). Dyslexia friendly schools in the UK. *Topics in Language Disorders, 26*(2), 144–156.

Ridsdale, J. (2004). Dyslexia and self-esteem. In M. Turner & J. Rack (Eds.), *The study of dyslexia* (pp. 249–273). New York, NY: Kluwer Academic.

Ritchie, S. J., Della Salla, S., & McIntosh, R. D. (2011). Colored overlays do not alleviate reading difficulties. *Pediatrics, 128*(4), E392–E398.

Roberts, T. A., Christo, C., & Shefelbine, J. A. (2011). Word recognition. In M. L. Kamil, P. D. Pearson, E. B. Moje, & P. P. Afflerbach (Eds.), *Handbook of reading research* (Vol. 4, pp. 229–258). New York, NY: Routledge.

Roper, H. D. (1984). *Spelling, word recognition and phonemic awareness among first grade students.* Unpublished doctoral dissertation, University of Texas, Austin, TX.

Rowan, L. (2010). Learning with dyslexia in secondary school in New Zealand: What can we learn from students' past experiences? *Australian Journal of Learning Difficulties, 15*(1), 71–79.

Roy-Charland, A., Saint-Aubin, J., & Evans, M. J. (2007). Eye movements in shared book reading with children from K to grade 4. *Reading and Writing, 20,* 909–931.

Samuels, S. J. (1979). The method of repeated readings. *The Reading Teacher, 32,* 403–408.

Scanlon, D. M., Gelheizer, L. M., Vellutino, F. R., Schatschneider, C., & Sweeney, J. M. (2008). Reducing the incidence of early reading difficulties: Professional development for classroom teachers versus direct interventions for children. *Learning and Individual Differences, 18,* 346–359.

Schonell, F. J. (1950). *Diagnostic and attainment testing: Including a manual of tests, their nature, use, recording and interpretation.* Edinburgh, UK: Oliver & Boyd.

References

Schonell, F. J. & Schonell, F. E. (1960). *Diagnostic and attainment testing* (8th ed.). Edinburgh, UK: Oliver & Boyd.

Seidenberg, M. (2013). The science of reading and its implications. *Language Learning and Development*, 9(4), 331–360.

Sénéchal, M., Ouellette, G., Pagan, S., Lever, R. (2011). The role of invented spelling on learning to read in low-phoneme awareness kindergartens: A randomized-control-trial study. *Reading and Writing*, 25, 917–934.

Shany, M. T., & Biemiller, A. (1995). Assisted reading practice: Effects on performance for poor readers in grades 3 and 4. *Reading Research Quarterly*, 30, 382–395.

Shavelson, R. J., & Bolus, R. (1982). Self-concept: The interplay of theory and methods. *Journal of Educational Psychology*, 74, 3–17.

Shaywitz, S. E. (1996). Dyslexia. *Scientific American*, 275, 78–84.

Shaywitz, S. E. (2003). *Overcoming dyslexia: A new and complete science-based program for reading problems at any level*. New York, NY: Alfred A. Knopf.

Shaywitz, S. E., Morris, R., & Shaywitz, B. A. (2008). The education of dyslexic children from childhood to adulthood. *Annual Review of Psychology*, 59, 451–475.

Singleton, C. (2005). Dyslexia and oral reading errors. *Journal of Research in Reading*, 28(1), 4–14

Snowling, M. J., Stothard, S. E., & McLean, J. (1996). *Graded Non-Word Reading Test*. Bury St., Edmonds, England: Thames Valley Test.

Stanback, M. L. (1992). Syllable and rime patterns for teaching reading: Analysis of a frequency-based vocabulary of 17,602 words. *Annals of Dyslexia*, 42, 196–221.

Stanovich, K. E. (1986). Matthew effects in reading: Some consequences of individual differences in the acquisition of literacy. *Reading Research Quarterly*, 21, 360–407.

Stanovich, K. E. (1996). Toward a more inclusive definition of dyslexia. *Dyslexia*, 2(3), 154–166.

Stanovich, K. E. (2000). *Progress in understanding reading: Scientific foundations and new frontiers*. New York, NY: Guilford Press.

Stephenson, J., & Wheldall, K. (2008). Miracles take a little longer: Science, commercialisation, and the Dore program. *Australasian Journal of Special Education*, 32(1), 67–82.

Sternberg, R. J., & Williams, W. M. (2010). *Educational psychology*. Upper Saddle River, NJ: Pearson.

Therrien, W. J. (2004). Fluency and comprehension gains as a result of repeated reading: A meta-analysis. *Remedial and Special Education*, 25(4), 252–261.

Thomson, P. (2004). Stress factors in early education. In T. R. Miles (Ed.), *Dyslexia and stress* (pp. 3–19). London, UK: Whurr.

Torgesen, J. K. (2000). Individual differences in response to interventions in reading: The lingering problem of treatment resisters. *Learning Disabilities Research and Practice*, 15, 55–64.

Treiman, R. (1994). Sources of information used by beginning spellers. In G. D. Brown & N. C. Ellis (Eds.), *Handbook of spelling: Theory, process and intervention* (pp. 75–91). New York, NY: John Wiley.

Tresman, S., & Snowling, M. (2005). Dyslexia is not a myth. *Literacy Today*, December, 7.

Tse, L. (2011). *Can phonics instruction and big book readership in combination work better than on their own?* Unpublished doctoral dissertation, Massey University.

Tse, L., & Nicholson, T. (2014). The impact of a phonics-enhanced Big Book approach on the language and literacy skills of six-year-old pupils of different reading ability attending lower SES schools. *Frontiers in Psychology*. doi: 10.3389/fpsyg.2014.01222

Tunmer, W. E., & Chapman, J. (1995). *Invented spelling test*. Palmerston North: Massey University.

Tunmer, W., & Greaney, K. (2010). Defining dyslexia. *Journal of Learning Disabilities, 43*(3), 229–243.

Van Kuyk, T. (1995). *The effectiveness of coloured overlays in the remediation of reading disabilities: A controlled study*. Unpublished master's thesis, University of Auckland.

Vellutino, F. R., Fletcher, J. M., Snowling, M. J., & Scanlon, D. M. (2004). Specific reading disability (dyslexia): What have we learned in the past four decades? *Journal of Child Psychology and Psychiatry, 45*, 2–40.

Vellutino, F. R., Scanlon, D. M., Sipay, E. R., Small, S. G., Pratt, A., Chen, RS, et al. (1996). Cognitive profiles of difficult to remediate and readily remediated poor readers: Early intervention as a vehicle for distinguishing between cognitive and experiential deficits as basic causes of reading disability. *Journal of Educational Psychology, 88*(4), 601–638.

Wadlington, E., Jacob, S., & Bailey, S. (1996). Teaching students with dyslexia in the regular classroom. *Childhood Education, 73*(1), Fall, 2–5.

Wanzek, J., Al Otaiba, S., & Petscher, Y. (2014). Oral reading fluency development for children with emotional disturbance or learning disabilities. *Exceptional Children, 80*(2), 187–204.

Watts, Z., & Gardner, P. (2013). Is systematic phonics enough?: The benefit of intensive teaching of high frequency words (HFW) in a year one class. *International Journal of Primary, Elementary, and Early Years Education, 41*(1), 100–109.

Whitehead, R. (2007, December). Dyslexia: Socially misunderstood. *Literacy Today*, 8–9.

Widdowson, D. A., Moore, D. W., & Dixon, R. (1998). Engaging in recreational reading. In G. B. Thompson & T. Nicholson (Eds.), *Learning to read: Beyond phonics and whole language*. New York, NY: Teachers College Press.

Wilkinson, G. S. (2006). WRAT4: *Wide Range Achievement Test*. Lutz, FL: Psychological Assessment Resources.

Wilkinson, G. S., & Robertson, G. J. (2006). *Wide Range Achievement Test 4*. Lutz, FL: Psychological Assessment Resources.

Winkler, H., & Oliver, L. (2003a). *I got a D in salami*. New York, NY: Grosset & Dunlap.

Winkler, H., & Oliver, L. (2003b). *Niagra Falls, or does it?* New York: NY: Grosset & Dunlap.

Wiseley, L. (2010, 27 April). Henry Winkler brings inspirational message to the Benchmark School. *Delaware County News Network*. Retrieved from http://www.delconewsnetwork.com/articles/2010/04/27/ridley_town_talk/news/doc4bcdad0fa2337826740230.txt?viewmode=fullstory

Wolf, M. (2007). *Proust and the squid: The story and science of the reading brain*. New York, NY: Harper Collins.

Wyllie, R. E., & Durrell, D. D. (1970). Teaching vowels through phonograms. *Elementary English, 47*, 787–791.

Glossary

Alien words—pseudowords or non-words that skilled readers can usually pronounce correctly such as *kniffle*, *sarth*, and *chrism*, because they are phonologically regular, even though they have never seen them before.

Alphabetic principle—the understanding that words are composed of letters and that letters represent sounds. It is using letter-sound correspondences (or grapheme-phoneme) knowledge to pronounce written words.

Anglo-Saxon (Old English) words—those spoken by the Anglo-Saxon inhabitants of England and Scotland in the 5th to 12th centuries.

Big Book reading—a strategy where the teacher reads an enlarged copy of a book to a small group or to the class so that pupils can all see the print. The Big Book could be an enlarged PDF copy of the book shown on a screen or electronic whiteboard. The teacher uses the Big Book as an instructional tool to teach reading, explaining how to decipher print by pointing out letter features and punctuation, explaining illustrations and unfamiliar vocabulary, and discussing overall meaning of the text.

Cipher knowledge—refers to a systematic relationship between written and spoken language where phonemes are represented by graphemes. It is complex in English because there are 40 or more phonemes but only 26 letters—in addition the rules of the cipher are implicit in that we cannot explain to pupils how to say some phonemes in isolation, e.g., the "b" and "g" in "bag" become syllables "beh" and "geh" when we try to pronounce them, and the word comes out as "beh-a-geh". These are not the actual phonemes in the word and do not sound like the word—the rules of the cipher are also context dependent, e.g., the letter "c" can have the sound of /k/ or /s/ depending on the letters that follow it.

Consonant—is a sound produced with some constriction of the air stream (e.g., /s/, /m/) There are 21 English consonants.

CVC—a combination of consonant, vowel, and consonant to form a pronounceable unit of sound, as in "buf"—Anglo Saxon spelling patterns are variants of CVC such as VC, CVCe, CCVCC, etc.

Developmental delay—generally means when the child does not reach developmental milestones on time—in reading it is when a pupil is not reading at their age level but reading at a level that is similar to a younger, normally progressing reader.

Digraph (or digram)—refers to two letters to represent one sound. An example of a consonant digraph is "ch" to represent the /ch/ sound.

Distal—distant.

Dyslexia—comes from Greek and consists of two word parts: *dys* meaning difficulty; *lexia* meaning words. In its simplest form dyslexia means difficulty with words.

Ectopias—from Greek meaning out of place—in the brain, refers to bundles of neurons that have moved place.

fMRI—used to measure brain activity—it measures levels of oxygen in the blood—when the brain is active blood levels increase and fMRI technology detects this.

Greek layer of English—Greek words entered English during the Renaissance. Greek words are compounded (comprise two equal parts, such as the word dyslexia), and appear largely in scientific texts.

Ideas—are thoughts, plans, designs, schemes—they represent a message that the writer wants to convey—these ideas could be informational as in an expository text or they could be narrative as in writing a story.

Intervention comes from the Latin intervenire, meaning "to come between, interrupt." It is an action designed to have an effect on something—in education, this would usually mean an effect on learning or behaviour. An example of an educational intervention in reading is Reading Recovery.

Invented spelling—where the beginner speller uses letter names as approximations for the sounds in words, e.g., LADE for LADY, using the "ee" name of the vowel.

Language comprehension—see listening comprehension.

Glossary

Latin layer of English—consists of a Latin root (e.g., scribe; rupt, struct) and a prefix and or/suffix. Latin based words are more formal and are found in reading material of older children (approximately 9–10 years).

Lexical knowledge—refers to knowledge of exception words, that is, words where spellings are not systematic e.g., where "ach" in "yacht" refers to /o/, or "olo" in "colonel" refers to /er/, and includes polyphonic spelling patterns such as the "ea" in ""sea" and "bread".

Listening comprehension—the ability to understand spoken language and to understand written language when it is read aloud.

Matthew effects—refers to the idea that in reading (as in other areas of life), the rich get richer and the poor get poorer.

Morpheme—is the smallest unit of meaning in a word.

Morphology—the study of word meanings, how words are built up with morphemes, e.g., "s" is a plural morpheme in the word "cats"; "cat" is a single morpheme – the word "psychometric" consists of 3 morphemes, psycho (mind), metre (measure), ic (adjective form).

Neuroscience—scientific study of nervous system and how they affect behavior and learning.

Onset-rime—the onset is the consonant or consonants before the vowel in a syllable; the rime is the remainder of the syllable (e.g., for the word dog /d/ is the onset and /og/ is the rime; for stop /st/ is the onset and /op/ is the rime.

Phoneme—is the smallest unit of sound in a word. The word *hat* has three phonemes /h/ /a/ /t/.

Phonemic awareness—is a conscious awareness of the smallest unit of sound in a word and an ability to manipulate the sounds (e.g., delete the /h/ from *hat* and replace with the phoneme /p/ to get *pat*).

Phonics—is a teaching approach that teaches letter-sound (grapheme-phoneme) relationship rules.

Phonological awareness—is an awareness of the different levels of speech sounds. Phonological awareness is conscious awareness of syllables (e.g., that the word *dog* is one syllable and *rabbit* is two); onset and rime; and phonemes.

Phonograms—in teaching reading, it usually refers to a letter sequence that stands for a syllable – it is actually a rime in that it is the part of the word that produces the rhyme, e.g., -ake in "cake" – it is the VC or VCC or VVC or VCe part of the word.

Phonological dyslexia—a kind of dyslexia where you can read real words like "jazz" but not made up words like "maz".

Prefix—is a unit of meaning, or morpheme, that is attached to the beginning of a Anglo-Saxon word (e.g., *un*happy) or Latin root (*de*struct). *Pre-* means before.

Prosody—usually associated with reading fluency and refers to the ability to use punctuation to read orally with expression.

Proximal—near.

Reading—the ability to decipher and to understand written text.

Reading accuracy—is the ability to recognise words either through analogy (e.g., flight), decoding (e.g., fat, rabbit, student), or as words with irregular spellings "sight words" (e.g., choir, the).

Reading comprehension—is the ability to understand what is read.

Reading fluency, or automaticity—is the ability to read words with no noticeable mental effort. It is when the reader has mastered word recognition.

Reading Recovery—a short term intervention for 6-year-old children who are the lowest achieving after their first year of school.

Repeated reading—refers to a strategy used in schools to increase reading fluency where pupils read and re-read the same text.

Romance words—includes word derived from Latin and from languages that are descended from Latin such as Spanish, French, and Italian.

Self-concept—is your view of yourself as well as how you think about you attributes and abilities.

Self-efficacy—is how you feel about your potential to succeed in a particular situation.

Self-esteem—is how you feel about yourself.

Semantic—to do with meaning.

Simple view of reading (SVR)—is a model of reading that assumes reading is the product of decoding and language comprehension. Based on this formula there are four types of readers: good decoding and poor language comprehension; poor decoding and good language comprehension; poor decoding and language comprehension; good decoding and language comprehension.

Simple view of writing (SVW)—this is an extension of the simple view of reading (SVR) – whereas SVR assumes reading is composed of decoding and language comprehension, SVW assumes writing is composed of ideas and spelling. The model predicts that even with perfect spelling, you will not be able to write unless you have ideas. Likewise, even with perfect ideas, you will not be able to write unless you can spell.

Spelling—the ability to write alphabetic characters in a sequence that corresponds to the phonemes in a spoken word and that matches the conventional spelling as in a dictionary.

Suffix—is a morpheme added to the end of a word (e.g., sitt*ing*) or a Latin root (construc*tion*) that makes a new word. Adding a suffix changes the meaning or the grammatical function of the word changes.

Surface dyslexia—a type of dyslexia where it is hard to read exception words, e.g., words like "was" and "rough".

Sustained silent reading—refers to a strategy used in school where students read silently at a certain time each day. It is silent reading so that students can practise their reading skills to develop fluency.

Syllable—is a unit of speech that contains a vowel and (optionally) consonants before and/or after the vowel sound.

Syntax—the rules of word order in a language.

Treatment resisters—are students who participated in intervention programmes but did not respond very well.

Turtle talk—the strategy of stretching out the sounds in a word, saying the word slowly, to make the phonemes more salient to the listener, e.g., s-u-n.

Vowel—is a speech sound produced with very little constriction of the air stream.

Word recognition—the ability to recognise words correctly and with minimal mental effort.

Index

ABC books 20
alien words 61–69, 72, 175-177, 269
Anglo-Saxon words 6, 88-91, 99-103, 111, 113, 117-119, 126, 127, 198, 208-244
apps for reading 20, 147
assessment
  - alien words test 61–69, 177
  - alphabet Test 178–180
  - British Picture Vocabulary Scale (BPVS) 71
  - Bryant Test of Basic Decoding Skills 175–177
  - Burt Word Reading Test 71, 100, 101, 106, 108, 114, 115
  - exemplars of writing 72
  - Graded Non Word Reading Test 72
  - listening comprehension 70
  - Martin and Pratt Non Word Reading Test 72
  - Neale Analysis of Reading Ability 70, 71, 82, 100, 106, 108, 114, 115,
  - Peabody Picture Vocabulary Test (PPVT) 16, 70, 100
  - Phonemic Awareness Test (GKR) 181–184
  - PRETOS – Proof reading Tests of Spelling 73
  - PROBE 69, 70, 71
  - Progressive Achievement Tests 69, 73
  - reading comprehension 69–72
  - running records 69, 71
  - Schonell reading and spelling tests 73, 99, 100, 101, 106, 108, 114
  - STAR Test of Reading Ability 69, 70,
  - Test of Basic Decoding Skills 175–177
  - Test of Early Written language (TEWL) 73,
  - Test of Written Language (TOWL) 72

behaviour issues 16, 25, 37–46
Big Book reading 145, 163
  - lessons for reading and spelling 251–256
books with phonemic awareness rimes and alliteration 75, 130, 131, 251
case studies
  - Ryan 100
  - William 106
  - Jade 115
cipher knowledge 124, 125
comprehension strategies 92
  - activating background knowledge 94
  - questioning 94
  - analysing text structure 94
  - creating mental images 98
  - summarising 99
CVC pattern 105, 117, 126
decoding lesson plans
  - short *e* vowel 188
  - *y* consonant 191
  - *st* blend 193
  - long *i* vowel 195
dot-to-dot phonics 202
Dyslexia
  - debate about 16
  - definition of 11–21, 30, 270
  - developmental delay 270
  - distal indicators 11, 13, 15, 19, 21
  - ectopias 13, 270
  - fMRI 13, 270
  - learning styles 24
  - phonological dyslexia 14, 281

- proximal causes 15, 165
- surface dyslexia 14

dyslexia-friendly classrooms 157, 159

fluency 6, 104, 139–147
- prosodic cues 141, 145
- speed of reading 140
- repeated reading 142
- sustained silent reading 143

Fry's common words 187

Greek words 126, 127, 248, 270

invented spelling 56, 100, 123–126, 183, 270

layers of English 86, 88, 91, 117

Matthew effects 81–84, 271

metacognitive strategies 40

model of learning to read 53

model of learning to write 54

morphology 126, 127, 271

Ms Nickleby's classroom 58–60

neuroscience 11, 13, 15, 23

parents 20, 147, 164, 165

phonemic awareness 20, 25, 54, 74, 87, 119, 181, 201

phonological awareness 18, 82, 86, 87, 91, 117, 271,

phonics 17, 19, 20, 50, 58, 145–147, 202, 203, 251

phonics strips 201

phonograms 130, 131, 203–205, 272

prosody 141, 272

Reading Recovery 3, 25, 146, 272

Romance words 91, 126, 127, 190

seating arrangements 151, 152

secondary classroom 155

self-concept 38–41, 272

self-efficacy 41, 272

self-esteem 33, 35, 37–46

semantic 19, 130

simple view of reading (SVR) 50–52, 273

simple view of writing (SVW) 52–53, 273

spelling
- lexical knowledge 55, 56, 271
- cipher spelling 55, 56, 124, 125
- cue spelling 124
- definition 123
- invented spelling 56, 124–126
- irregular spellings 14, 55, 71, 125
- lists for learning to spell 131, 151
- phases in learning 123
- sample spelling lessons 208–244
- semantic relatives for spelling 130
- sound boxes 128, 204, 205, 208
- strategies 121–131
- teaching 122

stress 151

syllables 69, 86–89

syllable lesson plan (open and closed) 89

syntax 273

treatment resisters 85–86, 273

turtle talk 128, 201–202, 252-256

tutoring programmes 80–81

vocabulary strategies 99

word recognition 146, 273

writing 131–137

www.ingramcontent.com/pod-product-compliance
Lightning Source LLC
Chambersburg PA
CBHW051147290426
44108CB00019B/2640